INSIDE THE WHITE COAT

An Insider's Guide About What to Expect, and How to

Succeed in Medical School

By Alan Schalscha and David Hume

Paperback: ISBN 978-1-7354800-0-8

Ebook: ISBN 978-1-7354800-2-2

Inside the White Coat

An insider's guide about what to expect, and how to succeed in medical school

Table of Contents

Dedication

During college, I managed a 27-floor dormitory and what I witnessed during my time as resident director was both enlightening and horrifying. When returning home for visits and sharing my stories over dinner, my mom would often say to me, "Write that down, as you may not remember later." After graduating from the University of Texas with a degree in Anthropology, I decided to travel to Guatemala. I first lived with a local family, and then I moved into an area orphanage. I would often send letters home filled with stories from my time abroad and when my parents would write back, there was always a note from my mom that said, "Honey, Please keep track of all of your experiences, as you may not remember them later." Upon returning to the U.S. I taught at inner city high schools in both Houston and Dallas. Some of the most valuable life skills and lessons I have learned came from those experiences. When relaying the heartwarming or heart wrenching tales from my classroom to my parents, my mom would often say, "Be sure to write that down". I heard the same thing while attending graduate school, then medical school, and again in residency. Then later, when I relayed stories of teaching in a medical school environment, I once again was instructed to, "Write it all down". My parents are now older and have some health challenges. My spouse and I have moved them in with us in an attempt to spend more time with them and to help where we can.

Mom and Dad, this is for you, and I have written it down.

- Alan

Purpose

What is the purpose of this book?

Why should you read it?

I vividly remember my attempts to gain information as related to a career in medicine. I recall the efforts made to glean insight into the good, the bad and the ugly of healthcare professions. Once, my dad referred me to a friend-of-a-friend who had a brother in the medical field in a roundabout attempt to help provide me with a purview into medicine (this really happened). I wanted to know how to prepare for medical school, how to decide on a specific specialty, and what life would be like before, during, and after medical training. I wanted to know what was the cost of medical education, and how or if I could afford it. I was unsure about the things I should be worried about, and worried that there was a strong chance that I was stressed about the wrong things.

This book serves as our attempt to answer some of these questions without the awkwardness of asking uninformed questions to complete strangers. It should serve as an initial guide to prompt you all to ask more specific questions later. Think of it as a buffet of general medical education information. While we hope reading this book will leave you better informed than you were prior to finishing our text, it will not serve as a complete meal/resource in any one area. As with any buffet, you may choose to later seek more of one thing and less of another based upon your knowledge or interest. We have included topics within our narrative focused on: 1.) what we think will be helpful, 2.) what we feel is important, and 3.) what we feel may be entertaining in an effort to both instruct and show the personal side of medicine. We hope you learn from us and leave this reading with the ability to better direct future inquiries. We also hope you do a bit of laughing.

I refer to "we" as there were two of us who provided the information for the text that follows. David Hume and I have been friends and colleagues since 1999 when we met as first year medical students. As related to sharing healthcare specific information, we have many similarities and also significant areas in which we each have our own strengths. Dave has always had an interest in finance and has developed expertise related to money management for healthcare professionals. He will share some of his wisdom within the second half of this narrative. I will offer more of my personal experiences to help you understand the people you will encounter and the processes you are likely to engage in while in medical school. We have also included our CVs at the end of the book to help illustrate our histories and experience and to help give credence to what we state in the text. We wrote this book because we have been where you are, and we want to help you get to the next stage more easily.

CULTURE OF MEDICINE

Is Now a Good Time to Enter the Medical Field?

Recently, I met with a group of student athletes from the University of Texas at Austin. They had put together a "pre-med club" and were both eager and anxious to explore careers in medicine. Some of them were certain they wanted to attend medical school, while others were exploring various alternative healthcare opportunities. They were all passionate advocates for their fellow human beings, but had heard of various "challenges" that exist in current day medicine. For those who knew healthcare professionals, they had been warned that this is NOT the opportune time to enter medicine. In fact, some of them were strongly encouraged to consider other career opportunities.

I listened to their thoughts and concerns and after a bit of reflection shared some of my experiences with them. I energetically stated, that *this is the perfect time to enter medicine!* The reasons to become a healthcare provider now are because of the challenges cited, rather than in spite of them.

Let me explain.

I believe we are in a transitional period in the United States as related to healthcare. *Fortune* magazine[1] reported that in 2018 the US spent $3.65 trillion on healthcare, representing about $11,212 per person, with 59% of that going to hospitals, doctors and clinical services. They found that private health insurance spending per person rose 4.5% between 2017 and 2018 even though the number of people enrolled remained the same. While we spend more than anyone else worldwide, we rank 27th in levels of health care. Our current system is inundated with inefficiencies. For

---

[1] Sherman, E. U.S. Health Care Costs Skyrocketed to $3.65 Trillion in 2018. Fortune.com. Published February 21, 2019. http://fortune.com/2019/02/21/us-health-care-costs-2/

example, some of the methods by which we provide care are based on the potential for medical liability. It is, sadly, not solely based on an evidence-based approach to care. What I mean by this is that providers make procedural decisions that will cover their risk for liability. For instance, we may order a diagnostic test to ensure that we aren't missing something, even if the evidence (patient history and physical exam results) does not point to a potential finding. This may seem senseless, but when you are the one carrying the legal risk as a care provider you, too, may be motivated to order a test that carries a low yield. This is merely one example of the ways in which our current culture adds to the waste within our system.

We are also in the midst of an electronic health record (EHR) evolution. Most care systems have transitioned from paper charts to utilizing electronic ones. In theory, this is an advancement in healthcare as it makes the care note legible, creates standardization in record keeping, and allows us to gather data and utilize data driven dashboards to make information-driven and population-based decisions. Today, I can place an order in the health record for a data retrieval that tells me which of my patients with diabetes are out of compliance. This in turn will allow me to reach out to those patients and manage their care more proactively. This approach would help me keep more folks in an active care cycle, thus decreasing the risk of diabetic downstream ramifications such as amputations, heart attacks, etc. These electronic records should also be able to communicate with other like systems so that regardless of whether a patient is in an in-house setting (in a hospital) or in an outpatient setting (primary or specialty care clinic), their care providers can know what has happened in the other environment and what the requisite follow up should be. This once again could help us with the patient's continuity of care. While we do have a legible record, we have not yet developed uniformity among EHR systems to where there is an active exchange of data between disparate systems. Thus, the silos that once existed, often still do.

While the implementation of EHRs has the potential to improve patient care, it is not a perfect solution. We have created unique reporting protocols for providers to ensure we can accurately retrieve the aforementioned patient data. When providers used to chart on paper, they were able to have a conversation with their patients and denote those conversations in a medical format directly into the chart. Though it took years of training to enable the provider to take a normal conversation and turn it into functional medical information, it was eventually able to be recorded on the patient chart in a linear fashion as the conversation occurred. Our need to collect and organize data requires today's providers to enter that data in specific fields (to make it searchable). This creates an asynchronous approach to care to where a physician now may have to chart on a different page, enter a piece of information and then return to where he/she was previously charting. This happens repeatedly, and the act of charting may now take much longer and that linear approach of having a conversation has now been interrupted. In addition, the conversation that used to occur through direct eye contact is now occurring with the providers face buried in the EHR on a computer as he/she enters the requisite data. This increases the charting time but does not necessarily improve the care of patients. Also, we have not reduced the number of patients that providers need to see in order to cover same overhead costs that have continued to exist and escalate. Thus, providers are spending more time charting even if they see the same number of patients as before. This additional time charting often occurs after hours for many providers, resulting in them spending less time with their families and friends. This additional workload is one reason for increased provider burnout.

With the increase in obesity and cancer trends in the US[2], and the medical complications that are associated with these ailments and

---

[2] Raghupathi W, Raghupathi V. An Empirical Study of Chronic Diseases in the United States: A Visual Analytics Approach. *Int J Environ Res Public Health*. 2018;15(3):431. Published 2018 Mar 1. doi:10.3390/ijerph15030431 (https://www.ncbi.nlm.nih.gov/pmc/articles/PMC5876976/)

other chronic diseases, patients are becoming more complex, not less. Yet, once again, we have not reduced the number of patients that our providers need to see. We are also now in the era of "value-based care". This is a care paradigm where we look at improving the quality of patient care and their healthcare outcomes. Though this is the direction that we as a nation are trending, we have not yet transitioned from a fee for service model (you bill for the number of patients you see and what you do for those patients) to a value based approach where you get paid for the quality (patient outcomes) of care you deliver. We currently expect providers to do both at the same time: see more patients and improve the quality of care they deliver to each one. Yet, we are doing that on an inefficient system that requires more time.

Another challenge in medicine today is the nationwide shortage of providers. This is especially true of primary care physicians[3], but remains a truism for almost every care specialty. Thus, creative approaches to care must be entertained. We are starting to utilize behavioral health therapists, dietitians, pharmacists, and other collaborative care team members to more actively manage patients in a team-based environment. This allows for much greater patient advocacy, increased access to care and a multispecialty approach. Still, we have not determined a payment methodology to support this model. The majority of insurance payers do not reimburse for visits with the other, non-M.D. /D.O. team members mentioned. We could also be utilizing our nursing and medical assistant staff to conduct blood pressure checks and to follow up on diagnostic exams and referrals, yet there is no reimbursement for these visits/interactions either. Thus, we (physicians) are bringing patients back into the clinic to gather/share basic information that could be done by other team

---

[3] New Findings Confirm Predictions on Physician Shortage. AAAMC.Org. Published 2019 April 23.
https://news.aamc.org/press-releases/article/workforce_report_shortage_04112018/

members, again utilizing an inefficient methodology and increasing overall costs.

For years, medical providers have been empaneled solely based on a set number of patients. In our system, for example, a full-time family medicine doctor carries a patient panel of 1,250 patients. We calculate panel size by looking at the available slots per day, number of days per year during which the clinic is open and the number of times an average patient should return to see the family doctor per year, which is about three times annually. This empanelment theoretically allows patients' access to their provider and allows the provider to get to know his or her patients in order to better improve their health. However, due to the need to continuously provide access for patients to care (too many patients and not enough providers), we tend to over empanel our providers, so they actively care for more than the prescribed 1,250 unique patients in their panel. This decreases the availability for each patient to return to the provider multiple times each year because those slots are filled with other patients. Simultaneously, it makes it tougher for the providers to improve patients care due to a reduction in opportunities to learn more about their patients' overall health. We currently hold providers accountable for objective outcomes; and though we have over empaneled them, we expect them to improve the objective metrics for each patient's specific disease. Yet another reason for provider burnout.

Now, consider the severity of disease burden. Each panel of 1,250 patients is not equal in disease complexity. Physician A's patients may be sicker than Physician B's patients, making the patient load heavier for Physician A. It takes longer to care for more complex patients. Health risk assessments could be critical to balancing physician patient panels. We should be decreasing the panel size for our providers who carry a more advanced panel (to allow them to spend appropriate amounts of time with each patient and improve patient care), while increasing the number of patients a provider is responsible for if they carry a less complex patient load.

Nevertheless, our current system has not done this balancing of the scales.

I stated at the start of this chapter that this is a time of transition in the medical field, and thus, it is the perfect time to enter a healthcare profession. There are many dynamic and intelligent people working daily on improving our current system. Still, we need more independent thinkers—those who are tech-savvy and mission-driven—who will provide different perspectives to advance our care model. If utilizing creativity, solving cognitive challenges, working on a team, and improving the health of others are aspects that energize you, then please go into medicine. In a decade, healthcare will look very different from the system we have today. Robert F. Kennedy once stated, "Only those who dare to fail greatly can ever achieve greatly". While this may be a bit dramatic as related to the current state of medicine in America, it does set the stage for utilizing our past efforts at care design to improve our future. Help us rethink and redesign the way by which we care for our communities. We need YOU.

A few months ago when I wrote the section above, COVID-19 was not a part of our daily culture. I feel it is important to share some of the clinical environmental changes as it speaks directly to what I delineated previously.

The first cases of this novel coronavirus presented in China in December of 2019. From that point, it rapidly spread around the world. COVID-19 officially entered the Austin community in late February and I remember we had to rapidly adapt to the "new normal" by Mid-March of 2020. This was about the time that Governor Abbott issued the stay at home order for Texans, and communities rapidly changed their daily routines. Schools were closed, only essential businesses remained open and many individuals began working from home. At the same time, ambulatory medical care institutions needed to decide what care was critical, what was not and how to administer both aspects. We created a war room and our operational/nursing and clinical teams came together in an effort to institute new clinical protocols. We are a large ambulatory system and care for around 2,000 patients a day. Within 4 days, our teams transitioned from an all in person model to 70% of our care being conducted remotely, both by way of video and telephonic visits. Protocols and processes that had been inefficient for decades and that I spoke of previously in this essay changed overnight. Yes, there were and are challenges with the new system of care delivery. That being said, mission driven, smart and creative individuals worked together with an inspirational drive to meet the patients where they were. By rapidly delineating a new model of care, our teams were able to continue to advocate for the health and wellbeing of our patients in a safe and more efficient environment.

The proverbial ball has started rolling; we need you to keep it moving.

GOOD PRACTICE

Practice Kindness

"Be kind whenever possible. It is always possible". - Dalai Lama

To succeed in medicine and in life, two behaviors are critical: this first is to be good to everyone you meet, and the second is to work hard. Medicine is as much about relationships as it is about knowledge. We have all witnessed really smart providers with a poor bedside manner and how that impacts patient care. It not only affects what people think of that provider, it also affects patient health progress. Dr. Bernie Siegel wrote <u>Love, Medicine and Miracles</u> in which he tells of his personal journey and lessons learned as he changed his approach to patients. His interpersonal communication with patients and his collaborative approach to care positively affected outcomes in surgery. This is an extreme example, but if being nice can improve surgical outcomes, think about how much it can affect all other areas within health care.

In today's clinical environment, we practice medicine as a team. Forming good relationships with your team will decrease the amount of work you need to do as an individual to advance your patient's care and it will increase the quality of the care conducted by the group as a whole. When medical students enter the hospital environment for the first time, you will very rapidly learn that there is a difference between textbook medicine and what exists in reality. When I began my clinical rotations, I quickly understood that experienced hospital nurses had a depth of knowledge that was inspiring. They knew how the hospital operated and they understood the nuances in patient care that years of bedside practice had taught them. Forming a respectful and professional relationship with the nurses on my team helped me advance in ways that studying the current recommended evidence-based approaches to care could not. As our relationships strengthened, the nursing staff began to look out for me. They paged me less in the middle of the night, and they went out of their way to call me when there was something unique or interesting to learn.

There are medical students, residents and doctors who feel and act superior to other members of the team. Please understand that your chosen field in healthcare does not make you smarter than those who work in different areas. It is even more important to grasp that while you are in the process of training, having egotistical approach to learning or possessing a sense of entitlement will make your daily work so much tougher and less enjoyable for you. When I was a resident, I really did not like wearing my white coat and often did not. I am bald and bulky and was often stereotyped to be an orderly. I have been asked to empty bed pans, clear food trays, and get additional blankets. I always helped out and never said, "I am a doctor, let me get the nurse". This earned me respect within the hospital, which I believe served me well throughout my training. Now, it is important to share that I did not let my "doctor" duties wane as this was my primary responsibility. Understanding how orderlies were treated helped me to reinforce the practice of humility, and respecting my peers (be they nurses, orderlies, or attendings) helped me to practice being kind.

Practice Looking Good

Appearance is important. Conservative dress may help you to avoid potentially offending the sensibilities of the dynamic populations you will engage with. You should also practice good grooming. You need to be showered, shaved (if applicable), and have your "office attire" ironed/pressed. When in clinic, I wear scrubs and they are always neat and clean. I am very comfortable in them and tend to load up my pockets with "stuff" which facilitates my patient care. When you are on service, ask about clinic protocol regarding dress and do not assume that scrubs are acceptable attire. The same is to be said of wearing your white coat—just follow protocol. Your goal should be to blend into the clinic culture, not to create a new one.

Closed-toe shoes may not always be the most fashionable, but they are the most practical and appropriate shoes for the clinical environment. Wearing shoes that cover your toes will protect you from falling medical instruments and/or bodily fluids landing on your toes or gently flowing between them (neither of which are crowd pleasers). There is also a risk of accidental needle stick if you have exposed feet. So, protect yourself (and your feet). While I understand the glove shoes are comfortable, they are not standard, not widely accepted, don't have a solid top and to be honest they just freak people out....so don't wear them. Wearing shoes that increase the longevity of your feet (shoes that are comfortable and supportive) while also being protective will serve you best.

Practice True Intentions

I have often wished that I had the opportunity to speak to more individuals before they entered the medical field. I would love to hear their reasons for wanting to become a nurse, a physical therapist or a physician. I have interviewed many medical student applicants over the course of my career, and I have heard their many reasons for applying. When in a formal interview, most answers are rehearsed; it is rare to be able to have a spontaneous heart-to-heart conversation with the interviewee. During those interviews all applicants speak of being mission-driven and of wanting to help humanity in a small or large way. Many interviewees state that they have had experiences, personally or through a family member or friend, that has motivated them to become a healthcare professional in order to affect positive change. I always hope that the stories I hear are true. I have learned, if applicants are not honest with themselves from the beginning, the journey to medicine is going to be that much tougher. I call this self-honesty "true intent". If a medical student applicant truly wants to enter the medical field because they want to help people, they like academic and physical challenges, and they enjoy teamwork, then I welcome them to medicine. If they are entering because their parent is in healthcare and that expectation has been passed down, or they want to earn a high salary, etc., it is going to be a tough road to travel.

A medical student who has true intent will most likely enjoy the journey more, put in more time, and stress less as their perspective on the process will have a more positive frame. This person will be inquisitive and may learn details that may not be on a board exam, but will render them a better doctor over the course of their career. A resident with true intent will check labs on a clinically tentative patient in the middle of the night, thus potentially avoiding a health crisis. That same resident will conduct a thorough physical exam on a hospital admission, even if it is 2 o'clock in the morning. This may include waking a patient up, removing clothing, and turning the patient over in order to be complete. This may seem like basic care, but there are some individuals who will neither take the time, nor devote the energy to be so comprehensive when they are fatigued. A healthcare professional with true intent will be a patient advocate regardless of the circumstances. We as attendings know very quickly which of our students are in medicine for the right reasons. Those students engage rapidly and are inspiring to teach. They add energy to the work environment and make our day/night better. They also take much better care of their patients.

Entering this field requires that individuals be honest with themselves about what it is they are embarking upon and what will motivate them when the journey gets tough.

Why are you wanting to enter medicine, what is your true intent?

Practice Confidence

(or fake it until you make it)

There is no life experience that prepares you for conducting your first rectal exam. There is no life experience that lays the groundwork for inserting a catheter (whether it's central or peripheral). There is no life experience that prepares you to use a scalpel on a live individual for the first time. Medical school serves as both the theoretical and functional training environment where these skills are learned. That being said, even when learning, there is a first time when a procedure will be conducted on a living person. It is for these situations that we tell our health professional students that they have to "fake it until they make it". More specifically, they have to inspire enough confidence to keep the patient on the exam table or in the chair in an effort to complete the procedure.

We need to be honest with patients, but there is a fine line between being brutally honest and opting not to share. Patients need to know that you are a student. They need to know that you are learning; they need to know you are being supervised. And, most importantly, they need to know the risks associated with the procedure being conducted. However, they do not need to know that this is the first time you have held a needle. They do not need to know that your heart rate is at 140 beats per minute. They do not need to know you have perspired through your undershirt; nor is it helpful for them to understand that you peed yourself just a bit in anticipation of the pending procedure. Your hands may be shaky as increased nervousness increases the upregulation of your sympathetic nervous system. Part of "faking it" means learning techniques ahead of time for hand stabilization and for calming yourself down. The most difficult aspect of most procedures is getting out of your own head. Try not to overthink it. If you are able to be calm and think through situations, you will be fine. The calmer and more thoughtful you are in your approach, the more opportunities you will be afforded to learn unique skills. After putting yourself in enough of those situations you will gain the confidence to know you can learn almost anything and the quality of your procedures will be better. Learn to be confident. A patient's ability to heal depends partly on you and their belief in you. Be confident, but don't be cocky. There is a fine line between the two and knowing the difference can make or break your career.

Practice Good Hygiene

I am writing this small section of text to address an act that: 1.) occurs with every patient encounter, 2.) is rarely considered, 3.) serves as the opening to patient care, and 4.) to entertain myself. I find it interesting to watch medical students, new to the clinical environment, as they enter the exam room. Hand washing is essential to good patient care, and any student who omits handwashing and/or using bactericidal gel between exam rooms increases the health risk to the patient and may not pass clinicals.

Now, the means in which this cleansing occurs within the care environment is often entertaining. What is best practice? Should a medical student enter the room, shake the patient's hand to introduce themselves and then proceed to wash their hands? This method makes for a smooth transition from the introductions, but there are patients that may wonder if the student doctor had soiled hands from their last patient encounter when they shook hands. Other times, many of patients will stand up as the student doctor enters the room to extend their hand for an introduction. If the student chooses to wash their hands before shaking the patient's hand, there is an uncomfortable dance between patient and student as the student professionally avoids all contact until they have washed their hands. Either method is correct, but many students get stuck between the two, which creates an awkward interplay between the patient and the medical student.

Ultimately, just remember to wash your hands (and try to avoid looking goofy).

Practice Being a Team Player

Teamwork is a big part of medical care and rounding is a prime example of how your perception and interplay with your teammates can and will affect your clinical experience. For example, if one of your fellow medical students is asked a question and they do not know the answer, do NOT automatically present the answer, unless asked to do so. If you volunteer information at the expense of a fellow teammate, well you have just voted yourself off the island. If the attending asks you, don't fake ignorance and state that you are unsure. In this case, you should present the information as known, but again don't volunteer it. Support your fellow team members and this will be repaid to you tenfold. Watch your body language if one of your teammates is struggling, don't be a silent jerk. Whether conducting hospital or ambulatory work, your ability to follow up for a colleague is critical to patient care. In addition, your teammates will also need to follow your patients, for example when you leave the hospital and the "on call" provider covers overnight. Being thorough in your patient care, completing your to-dos (checking diagnostics and placing orders) allows for your teammate to concentrate on new admissions or new results that need to be acted upon. Getting out of clinic early so that you can avoid traffic is not good for your patients nor your collaborative work relationships. Great friendships are forged in both medical school and residency, and some of those relationships are based on the respect we gain by watching how our colleagues advocate for patients.

Practice Self-Care

The first few months of medical school will feel like a whirlwind. However, once you make it to that fifth month, you will find that you have a slightly greater sense of familiarity with your routine. You can now identify every bookstore and coffee shop within a 5-mile radius of where you live by the stale coffee smell that resides on your collection of sweatshirts. You know The University of Texas sweatshirt with the holes in the sleeves and the fraying neckline was last worn at Pete's Coffee as the coffee smell there is slightly sweeter than that of The Coffee Bean. You have your favorite seat picked out in each java establishment and will have an almost visceral response whenever there is a "recreational" reader in your spot. Most study days require four cups of coffee, and you only remember to take a break and go home when the coffee shop closes around you.

Each night you attempt to fit in another hour of studying before your body becomes so fatigued that you must go to bed. Sleep comes restlessly, since your coffee habit negatively impacts your ability to snooze. Your morning alarm clock always rings too soon, and with its sound come thoughts about the six to eight hours of lecture that you will need to sit through today. The sitting itself does not concern you, but rather the additional information that will accumulate as the hours pass. Feeling behind at the start of the day stresses you out more than you can express. All of your free time is spent studying, and there does not seem to be time to merely chat with your friends and family. The friendships you are forming with your medical school peers still seem superficial; and ultimately, you feel very alone. You may begin to wonder why you are in medical school at all, and if it is possible that you are the only one who is struggling.

Each day progresses as it has for the past five months, and with each additional day comes a bit more dread and a slight depression. It takes more discipline to convince yourself to put in the prescribed four to five hours of study time daily after class. You are really now becoming fixated on the fact that you are suffering alone and feel isolated. How could you possibly be the only person having difficulty with the huge amount of information that needs to be memorized?

You are not alone. Let me say it again, it is NOT just you. Most of your classmates are similarly suffering and have the same symptoms as you. Many are crying their caffeinated selves to sleep, but will paint on smiles to make it through the day. It is important that when these thoughts and feelings arise, you reach out to your classmates and the school administration. You need to let others know of the struggles you are having and let them share their own difficulties and or assist you by getting help. Do not let medical school take your sanity. Your wellness is equally as important as your study time. So, remember to exercise! The endorphins help with the stress of school, and the physical activity helps to counter all the sitting you do while studying. Eat regularly and pay attention to your nutrition! A well-nourished body/mind actually improves memory and learning. And, I know it seems impossible, but you should make time to see your friends and family who are not in medical school with you. Spending some of your time with people that have a different life perspective can positively impact your happiness. I cannot explain how important these things are to your longitudinal health and well-being. And, remember, you need to take care of yourself so that you can one day take care of others.

CLINICAL ROUNDS

Taking a History

The patient history and physical exam serve as the foundation that enables the provider to then determine a diagnosis and treatment plan. The history (what the patient states) serves as the subjective portion of the exam and the physical (what you observe) serves as the objective portion.

When taking a history, an ideal patient will share with you why they have come in and everything that is significant to their ailment (from their perspective). The patient will most certainly provide this information in rapid coherent sentences that describe the onset of the problem, its location, duration, character (nature), the exacerbating and relieving factors and all other criteria associated with the reason for the visit. They will also share past medical, surgical, family and social history with you. Lastly, the patient will have a concise list of their medications, noting the medicine, its dosage, the frequency of usage and the mode by which it is taken. The patient will also deftly describe any allergies to past medication and how those allergies manifests themselves. Unfortunately, this will never happen. NEVER. There is a better chance of encountering a unicorn (these don't exist—don't tell my daughter) than this ever occurring. Rather, the patient will most likely provide you with a lengthy, yet insufficient, story that provides you with little useful information for diagnosing their concern.

The reality of the situation is your years of medical school and residency provide you with the basic tools needed to begin to understand the complexities of how we function as human beings. It will take years to fully learn what subjective information is critical to moving care forward and then what objective (the exam) information is needed to verify your pending assessment (diagnosis). There is a voluminous amount of information that you as the provider need to collect in a minute amount of time. You must gather it, synthesize it, and then utilize it to direct your exam, formulate a diagnosis, and create a plan for managing that diagnosis. For this reason, providers often interrupt patients every few seconds. We are trained to collect information in a systematic way so that we can be efficient and complete. We understand the processes better than our patients and we know what information is critical and what is not. For example, Mary may tell you about her pet dog, Spot, who used to be a Monday, Wednesday, Friday and every other Sunday stooler, but last pooped a week prior to today—which is atypical from the dogs usual stooling routine and this change has caused significant stress. The important aspect for us as providers is the increased stress the patient feels while the editorial that led to its reveal is not. Nevertheless, it is important to remember that nothing is absolute; there will be times when you will dismiss what a patient is telling you as insignificant and you will be wrong. There will also be times when you will include an aspect of the history that you thought tantamount to the eventual diagnosis and in hindsight it would have been of little use. Efficiency is key, and thus, you will frequently interrupt your patients.

The history is organized into multiple subheadings. First, it lists the chief complaint which is then followed by the history of present illness. The **Chief Complaint** is the reason for the patient's visit. It is usually stated in the words of the patient and we try to educate our nursing staff not to summate or draw a conclusions/make a diagnosis using the chief complaint. For example, if a patient presents to clinic for a sore throat, then the chief complaint is "sore throat" not "pharyngitis". The reason for avoiding rewording a patient's chief complaint and offering a summation term as a chief complaint is it may narrow your considerations for diagnoses. The final diagnosis for a patient with a chief complaint of sore throat may indeed be pharyngitis but it may also be reflux, postnasal drainage, a tonsillar abscess, sleep apnea, etc. all of which may cause a sore throat.

A personal note: I think it is unfortunate that over time we have referred to the reason for someone's visit as the "chief complaint". The reason I feel this way is patients often hear us speaking of them and we may state, "A 24-year-old male presents complaining of..." I am concerned that this verbiage may make the patients feel as though we think they are whining and thus affect what they tell us. Our profession requires us to be as objective as possible and this may in a very small way affect that. It is for this reason that I ask all providers presenting patients to state, "A 24-year-old male presents with...."

Following the chief complaint is the **History of Present Illness**—these are the details describing the chief complaint. This is normally organized into onset, location, duration, exacerbating and relieving factors and associated signs and symptoms. There are many pneumonic aids to help to learn this. These will help differentiate a heart attack from pneumonia and rib pain from reflux. The history of present illness is critical to understanding your patient. I often ask students what they feel is more important the history or the physical. Most students state that the physical is the key to making a correct diagnosis. Now obviously one should not live in isolation of the other. It is the history that provides the clues to the diagnosis and the physical that should serve to confirm that diagnosis. If you as a provider have completed the historical aspect of the workup and you have no idea what is going on with your patient, conduct a detailed physical but be very careful making an assessment. You may need to go back to the history and ask more questions. Your understanding of what is going on with your patient prior to hands on is critical to the well-being of your patient. This history is also conducted prior to the physical because it allows you to build rapport with your patient, hopefully developing a level of trust, before we actually touch them for the examination.

Presenting Patient Information

Presenting is a term that most frequently refers to the summation of the history and physical and the "presenting" of that information to your attending and/or the healthcare team. I cannot emphasize enough how important this skill set is. Your understanding of the patient and your ability to care for that patient will be evaluated within the first ten seconds of your presentation. In addition, the first presentation you deliver will most likely determine the course of your rotation. I know this does not seem like a very fair method by which to evaluate a medical student, so let me explain why it is done. Your patient presentation is really a summation of your data collection, your understanding of that data, the assessment of your patient and the plan you have formatted to advance patient care. If you are unable to present this in a predictable, well organized, and concise format, your attending will neither take the time to listen to you, nor entrust you with the care of their patients. Your attending does not have the luxury of time, so efficiency here is critical. Your presentation will either earn you grace and trust within your rotation or hang a big sign around your neck that states, "I am unsure of what I am doing so please let the pimping begin". Pimping when utilized in a medical teaching environment has to do with you being asked questions. Being questioned by those farther along than you are in their medical training is a part of our system of clinical learning. The anxiety that lives within all of us as we enter a new learning environment during training is almost palpable, as we know we will not be able to answer most of what is asked. This is why reading prior to changing environments benefits both you and ultimately your patients. Poor presentations loudly display your sparsity of knowledge and skill sets. Your presentation skill sets should have been mastered by the end of your second year in medical school and thus if you are having trouble during your third, fourth or during residency...as I said, let the pimping begin.

As a basic rule, if the story (your patient's history) does not make sense to you, it most certainly will not make sense to someone else. If there are aspects of your patient's history that are missing, go back and fill in that information by returning to speak to your patient, looking at old records etc., prior to presenting your patient to the team. Once you have organized the information, approach the presentation as you would a public speaking gig. If you read your entire presentation from the screen/paper, you will lose the engagement of your audience and it will appear that you do not know the subject matter. Part of your training will require you to have the history and physical template cemented in your cerebrum. Thus, when you meet with patients, you will just fill in the pertinent positives and negatives of their case. While presenting, you are welcome to refer to your H&P (history and physical notes), but do not read it verbatim. If you truly understand the patient's case, you should be able to tell the story without reading it. Answering questions about a specific patient will be easier when you talk about the patient from memory rather than read about your patient from your notes. Cognitively, you are already engaged at depth in this care and this makes answering questions easier.

I would also advise you not to summate or shortcut your presentation. If there are 100 attendings on staff at a hospital, you can guarantee there are 100 different preferences on how to present. While this seems like an impossible barrier to delivering a successful outcome, thoroughness and organization are your tickets to doing a good job. No attending has the time, nor patience to allow you to give a complete presentation on every patient-so you need not worry about this happening again. That being said, if you shortcut your first one, there are questions your attending will have that you have not answered in your summation and that will then beg the pimping protocol. A more thorough presentation also helps assure good patient care. For example, if at the beginning of your third year in medical school you are standing in front of your team presenting and have summated what you think is going on, you may have missed some random symptoms that did not seem relevant at the time but may actually point to a more comprehensive disease process. For example, if your patient comes in concerned about a cough and while you were working it up the patient stated that he experienced other symptoms. These are: shortness of breath at night when he lies down, some swelling in his lower legs, being more tired than normal, and not having the same energy he used to. This is a pretty good symptomatic description of heart failure, but the clues may seem like isolated symptoms and may not put together by someone new to medicine; whereas, a more experienced provider may connect the dots. Thus, you should present comprehensively in order to ensure that the patient receives the best care possible.

If during your presentation you are asked a question regarding your patient, or a general medical question and you do not know the answer, do NOT make one up. There are no gold stars for creativity here. If it takes more than two seconds for you to come up with an answer, you do not know it. The uncomfortable silence that exists between the time a question is posed and the time the answer is given is painful for everyone. Attendings will respect you saying you do not know the answer to the question. This should be followed up with, "I will research the answer and present it on rounds tomorrow". It is understood that if there is a gap in your knowledge base that is delineated while rounding, it is your responsibility to fill it prior to the next day. For example, if you are asked the pathophysiology of how a certain medication works, look it up that night and be ready to provide the information if asked the next day. A good tip here is to preview the information again before rounds the following day and ask the attending if you may answer the question that was asked yesterday. Taking this approach shows initiative on your part, not to mention you would have just read the information and it will be fresh in your mind. In contrast to this, if you wait for your attending to ask you about your assignment on the day prior, you are now being seen as reactive; and you may no longer have the information properly summated since new patient case data may have entered your brain since you last looked up the information.

Being on Call / First Night on Call

While in medical school, the idea of being "on call" is often viewed as appealing as it offers you a reason to brag. You may tell your friends that you cannot go out as your patient may deliver and you may be called in. You may wear your pager/carry your phone as a badge of honor frequently checking phantom pages in your passive-aggressive approach of informing your friends that your knowledge base is so great that you may be contacted just to answer questions. You may spend the night in a call room while covering with your attending or resident taking call once or even maybe seven times during your month on service. You will not hesitate to share this with family and friends as it means free passes for bad behavior, excuses to be freed from unwanted tasks and even a chance for special favors. However, please remind yourself that while on these rotations you will participate in patient care, many times significantly, but are not and should not be ultimately responsible for end point care. While you work incredibly hard in medical school, your on-call months will be limited, thus allowing you the chance to catch up on your lost sleep. You will also have someone there to help you with patient care, or rather, for you to help them with their patient care. It is important to understand that the smarter and more responsible you are, the more you will be trusted with patient care; but ultimately the care is the responsibility of the resident. This wonderful paradigm rapidly shifts when the resident is you.

I looked forward to being on-call since the beginning of medical school, and then dreaded it after my first call as an intern. I remember my official first day on call, as do my close friends: Dave and Dawn (name changed for privacy). We had all just graduated from medical school two months earlier. I was now in Albuquerque, NM; Dave was in Phoenix, AZ and Dawn was in Spokane, WA. Freakishly, we ended up being scheduled for our first call as interns on the same night. The three of us agreed that we would keep our phones on vibrate and pay special attention to them to serve as a lifeline for one another. There was a 30-hour rule in effect at that time. In theory, that meant that the most time we would spend in the hospital in one sitting was 30 hours.

The day began at about 6 o'clock on a Tuesday morning. I rounded on my patients, wrote my notes and presented at morning rounds. Afterward, I rounded with my attending, specific treatment protocols were discussed, and our patient care team dispersed to carry out these plans. There were two senior residents, three interns and three medical students on my team. I was efficient and could manage most of my patients' needs without too many questions directed to our senior residents. I worked closely with a medical student; together we completed most of the ordering for the diagnostic tests, labs and meds needed. We contacted specialists and discharged a patient as previously directed in rounds. We were close to completing our to-do list when the pager starting sounding. I want to advise you to choose the ring tone of your pager very carefully. In the future, any ring tone that even remotely mimics your pager from residency will cause an increased sphincter tone, rapid heart rate, some diaphoresis, mild nausea and an occasional vomiting.

Upon the first page we were notified that there were two patients in the emergency department (ED) that needed histories and physicals completed and orders dropped. This included any diagnostic tests that needed to be conducted both now and in the morning. It took an hour and a half to work both of the patients up. It was almost noon when we finished admitting the new patients, and I sent my medical student to go and grab some lunch. I still needed to complete my tasks from my own morning patients as I knew many of my fellow teammates were close to competing theirs and needed to check out for the day. Checking out required that each resident present their patients to me as the intern on call, and it was my responsibility to see to it that their patients' care continued to be carried out until rounds the next morning. My seven patients had grown to 15 as the other residents checked out.

By 2:30pm, I had still not eaten lunch. As all medical personnel know eating, peeing and sleeping only occur when there is a break in the action. So, lunch for me occurred at 2:30pm, during which I received another call from the ED with two more patients to admit. I finished my sandwich and drink in less than five minutes and then headed back to the emergency department. I asked my medical student to begin the workup on one of the patients while I admitted the other. We then presented to the attending and I sent the medical student home at about 5:30 that evening. I needed to go back upstairs to follow up on the multiple tasks delineated by the rest of my team. These tasks in addition to another ED admit took me until 10 o'clock that night to complete, when yogurt and an apple served as my dinner. I decided to get some sleep, but found myself only lying down from 10:05 pm to 10:30 pm. (Technically I closed my eyes, but the fear that I had forgotten to do something, fear of the pager going off, or of the pager not going off had me constantly checking it for messages. I also have to mention one of my least favorite aspects of sleeping in the call room was the pillow. The on-call pillow was a paper-like pillow cover snuggly fitted around a pillow that seemed to be wrapped in what looked like a plastic bag. This created incredible noise when moving one's head, not to mention it stuck to your face.)

Due to a combination of anxiety and needing to follow up on patients, I got off the bed and went back to the telemetry floor. Of note, you always get off the bed not out of it. This is because you never actually get in it—this would allow the unique fantasy of that sleep is an option. As I headed to the floor my personal phone buzzed, it was Dawn. I asked her how her day is going so far and heard both laughing and crying at the same time. She said she needed help STAT and would rapidly give me the scenario she was facing. I put on my game face and waited for her to present her patient so that I could share my wisdom. Dawn's need for assistance was much more critical than anything I could have imagined. It seemed that at about 10:30pm, she had gone to the restroom and due to her actions and lack of sound judgment was now suffering the consequences. As a medical student it is customary for each of us to wear a short white coat. Upon graduation and once we were all anointed the prestigious title of physician, we progress from a short white coat to a full-length coat. It appeared that Dawn was used to peeing with her white coat on and had forgotten that her previously short coat, was not so short anymore. Yes, she urinated on her coat and was calling her lifeline to find out what to do. She was still in the bathroom when she called me. Her name was embroidered on her coat; so simply leaving it there was not an option. I suggested she splash water all over it and create the facade that she is not good with faucets. She accepted my assessment and plan, calmed down and we both progressed with our day.

Four to five hours later, I was still caring for the team's patients but took a break to recharge. The ability to recharge was a bit of wisdom shared with me when I was a medical student, by a wise senior resident. I grabbed my overnight bag and headed to the men's restroom where I took out my contact lenses, washed my face, brushed my teeth and then... (wait for it) ... *changed my socks*. You would not believe how refreshed you will feel with a new pair of socks on. It seems decisions are made more easily, and tasks are completed more efficiently with clean, dry socks. I then began rounding on my patients at about 6am and then repeated my routine from 24 hours prior. I did take a break before morning rounds for eggs, bacon and hash-browns which were smothered in Aunt Cholula sauce. To be honest, breakfast was always the motivating force that allowed me to make it through most calls. Once rounds were completed, I checked out my patients, grabbed my overnight bag and headed for the parking garage. It was noon a day and a bit after I had started my shift. I had been in the hospital for 30 hours straight and could not wait to get home.

As I entered the parking garage Dave called. We had not spoken once during our night on-call, and it seemed like his night was much like mine. Dave, however, was more frustrated with the codes he needed for reporting than by complex patient care. He told me that he had patients on the phone but could not find his computer access codes for their floor. He needed to follow up on patient labs and imaging, but both systems required different sign-in methods. He stated that he had discharged a patient and needed to complete the discharge summary but could not remember the telephone codes used to complete it. He said, "Schalscha, to be honest, if your number was not programmed in my phone, there is a good chance I would have forgotten how to call you". As I was listening to him, I realized that I had been walking around the parking garage for 30 minutes. Then it dawned on me: I had been in the hospital for so long that I had no idea where my car was. I was actually having trouble remembering what it looked like.

So, your first (or 50th) night on call can go like mine, or like Dawn's, or like Dave's. If nothing else, remember to program your codes into a password safe for easier recall, mind your white coat in the restroom, and pack fresh socks. With these tips, you'll be well on your way to survival.

Always Go First

Of course, I remember when we were taught how to conduct a rectal exam, who wouldn't? Yet, the reason for this visceral memory is not one you would expect. The "invasive" exam portions of our physical exam course occurred during my second year of medical school. We were divided into groups of four and then assigned to a standardized patient and an attending. The standardized patients were individuals from the community/actors who were being paid to function as teaching patients. Many of them have been doing this for years and they serve as an invaluable resource to gaining specific skills that would be difficult to learn and practice otherwise. We actually conduct either the prostatic or pelvic exams on these patients, but with their feedback and an attending providing live instruction.

To initiate the exam, my group entered the patient's room, and we introduced ourselves to both the patient and the preceptor. The patient was sitting in a chair wearing a gown that opened in the back. The teaching exam room was set up to mirror what would be seen in a primary care outpatient clinic setting. If you want to experience medical student humility, be present during one of these exams. I can tell you that all egotistical pretense vanishes when faced with the challenge of completing your initial rectal exam, especially when done in front of your peers. The attending asked if anyone wanted to volunteer to conduct the exam first. Everyone in my group avoided eye contact; we angled our heads down and tried to melt into the wall that we had been leaning against. Since none of us volunteered, the attending assigned us turns. I was lucky number three. The attending proceeded to explain how the procedure was done and why. The verbal instruction reinforced what we had previously reviewed in our readings. Medical student Number One then stepped up to bat. He progressed through the exam with some challenges. This was expected as he was the first to participate, thus there was no historical perspective to learn from. Number Two stepped up to conduct the exam. She did fairly well and made fewer mistakes than our classmate, but still struggled a bit. I was nervous to start, but as time lingered my anxiety increased. Now, it was my turn. I had heard the explanation of how and why to conduct the exam twice. I had the luxury of learning from my classmates' mistakes, and now I felt pressure to perform better than they had. My heart was beating so forcefully and rapidly; I could hear it in my ears. That day I completed my initial rectal exam. I consider the fact that I made it through a personal triumph. This was not due to my deftness of the procedure, but rather that it was now behind me, no pun intended. Thinking back, my goal that day was to avoid injuring myself or my patient and to simultaneously try not to embarrass myself in front of my classmates. I checked all three of those boxes, thus I consider it at least a triple in baseball analogies.

It was now time for Number Four to go and bat clean up. She had been remarkably quiet during the previous three exams. Looking at her now startled me; she did not appear well. The three of us who had previously gone, were standing against the wall facing the patient, maybe seven feet from the exam table. The patient, upon instruction from student doctor Number Four, traveled from the chair (where the consultation happened) to the exam table. The patient, let's call him Tom, was then asked to lay in the left lateral decubitus position (basically on his left side). Both the preceptor and Number Four were behind the patient and the preceptor was calling the play by play in an effort to walk her through the exam. Looking at Number Four, I noticed that her complexion was significantly different from earlier. She was a whitish green, which was a coloration I had not seen until that time. We watched as she lifted the gown of the patient, narrating what she was doing as she proceeded. This served to reinforce to the attending that she knew what she was doing and to educate and warn the patient of what, when, and why each step was happening. One of the unique techniques Number Four chose to engage was not to actually look at the focal area of the exam. We all watched in awe and apprehension as perspiration ran down Number Four's face and dripped to the floor. As her index finger blindly tried to find the edge of the rectum, we eagerly anticipated the moment that the gentle insertion would occur—we would all know as the distance to the prostate would cause Number Four to lean a bit forward. However, this did not occur quickly, and Number Four's finger seemed to be traveling far too great a distance between the patient's glutes, evidently not finding its way to the intended target. After what seemed like an eternity, we saw Number Four stop and move her arm slightly anteriorly (forward), the patient rocked forward slightly and his facial expression changed. Celebration for all, she had now found and entered the rectum. However, she had forgotten to continue to narrate her way through the exam and thus she appeared to have entered the rectum with too great a velocity not to mention this came as a surprise to the patient. The attending noticed this and so started to coach number 4 on the proper technique. She stopped what she was doing and listened to the attending, though kept her index finger where it was. The attending spent what seemed like a lifetime reviewing proper protocol. The entire time, Number Four's finger was buried deep within the patient. The patient looked at the rest of us with both amazement and concern. His face did not resemble pain, but rather confusion. It took all the self-control we could muster not to laugh out load. During all of this, the finger continued to be stationary. It was then that we then saw Number Four turn one shade greener. Through her white coat we saw an abdominal heave, followed by her shoulders elevating and we are all positive she would vomit on Tom. She somehow held it in, but I am certain that she vomited in her mouth. Finally, it was over. Number Four did not hit a home run, but eventually she did complete the exam. Two years later when she graduated, she chose pediatrics as a specialty—we think this is most likely due to PEDS not requiring rectal exams.

So, what can we learn from the interaction between the 4 of us and our patient, Tom? Always go first! Let me restate this, when there is any opportunity to volunteer, volunteer first and do it rapidly. There are no negatives in volunteering to serve as the preemptive guinea pig. It shows both initiative and courage. Waiting be chosen by your attending to go first does not earn you points for courage. Going first also means there is no precedent for you to live up to. If you don't do so well, you may be shown grace in your evaluation as there is no standard to compare you to. Do not worry that others will do better. Remember, by you going first, they will learn from your mistakes. Lastly, consider what your autonomics will do as you wait for your turn. More likely than not, increasing anxiety will cause you to perspire and shake as time accumulates.

Avoid experiences like Number Four's. Always go first.

Mind the Hierarchy

It is important to understand that a medical hierarchy exists and that it is as old as medicine itself. This hierarchy serves to organize patient care, aids to ensure that appropriate oversight is provided while conducting care, and lets you know to whom and for whom you are responsible. It is vital to recognize the existence, and to understand the purpose and the limitations of this hierarchy.

Medical education is unique in many aspects. Due to its concentrated nature and steep learning curve, one year between educational/experiential levels is vastly different from the next. Learn the functionality of the hierarchy and your place in it. Those more advanced in the process (senior medical students, interns, residents) really should know more information and should serve to guide those with less experience. Look to your seniors for mentorship, not competition.

As a general rule, under-speak and over-produce. If you are unsure of whether certain patient information should be shared with the team, run it by your senior for advisement. Realize that you are an extension of the person who is responsible for you and thus any incorrect or ill-prepared patient care reflects directly on them. Do not over-speak your attending. It is really important to understand that when you are sent into an exam room, you are the physician representative and the director of patient data collection and health care maintenance. It is even more important to understand that the moment the attending is in the room, you are a passive observer, unless directed otherwise. If you enter a room together, make sure you allow the attending to interview the patient and ask all of the questions. Also, make sure they are the one to provide all of the answers to the patient and staff questions. There are many times that attendings will not ask questions as they may already know the answers, or they will ask them in a specific format to illicit specific information to help make a better diagnosis. It is both a sign of overconfidence and a lack of understanding if the student preempts the physician and doing so may have negative ramifications for you.

There seems to be a growing notion that physicians (and future doctors) are entitled to more. Please realize that we are not. Life is not fair. No one cares how hard you have worked and what you have sacrificed in the past. Most likely the person standing next to you has worked harder and sacrificed more to get to the same place. You should let the past motivate you; and a strong work ethic advance your own future. Looking at the past as entitling you to a certain future is not beneficial and will alienate many of your team members along the way.

Supervisors Are Not Always Mentors

I wish I could tell you that the people ahead of you in the educational process are smarter, more compassionate and generally wiser than you are. The truth is that many of them are not. Many have struggled along the way, both learning their academic knowledge and mastering their clinical skills. There will also be a large group of individuals whose life experience will be limited.

Meet Dr. Awkwardness, your attending. He is 28 years of old, an only child, single and has never had any hobbies or other interests other than medicine. He is not the brightest person in the room and he has no sense of humor. Due to his lack of both medical and non-medical skills, he is an insecure person and an average physician. He may not deal well with your charismatic personality as your patients may start directing their attention to you instead of him. He may not entertain your broad differential diagnoses since his are pretty limited, and his practice of medicine is based on what he has diagnosed in the past. He also may not be very empathetic towards the patients as he has no life experience to help him relate to them or properly council them. Thus, he may not speak to you much, may not ask you for your opinion, and may not compliment you when you perform well or encourage you when you do not. If you understand this going in, you will be fine. You can learn a ton from the worst physicians.

A note: It is worth saying that it is important to know the difference between someone not being "nice" to you and someone who is "inappropriate". If you ever feel you are being treated differently due to ethnicity, gender, age, sexual orientation, etc.—that is inappropriate. If your senior did not ask you what you had for breakfast and does not care what your hobbies are, it may not be nice, but it is not inappropriate. Know that you should never compromise who you are as a person, especially if it is based on an ignorant stereotype.

Many times in medicine, we learn what not to do, rather than what to do. It is neither ideal nor fun, but it happens. The important thing is that you are progressing as a medical student/learner. You need to understand that someone further along in this unique educational process is just that, further along. Do not define yourself by every bad comment or pieces of negative feedback that you receive. Learn from the criticism, but temper your emotional response by who is giving the feedback and why it is being given. There will be many times when you will think about throwing your overloaded white coat on the floor, verbally assaulting your attending, flinging the 13 pens you have in your pocket against the wall and leaving the clinic or hospital. It is for those moments that this passage is important. This bears repeating: do not reevaluate yourself as a person if you have a bad day or if your attending is a shmuck. Simply learn from it and move on.

Being Pimped

We have touched on this topic briefly before; however, because it is such a large part of the medical education culture, I think it is important to visit at greater depth. "Pimping" is a teaching style that utilizes an aggressive, rapid-fire style of Socratic questioning to test medical students' clinical knowledge. Pimping is typical for learners in the clinical setting, and often occurs in front of patients and peers.[4] I do not know what evidence-based studies state regarding teaching methods that involve the Socratic Method. Regardless of what they show, pimping exists in the medical classroom setting, in the hospital and in the clinic. There is no way to avoid it, thus understanding its nature and preparing for it is the best way to survive the experience.

I have had the luxury of lecturing to medical students for many years and it is really easy to identify students who are petrified of being called on. They avoid eye contact, constantly look down and shy away from any form of engagement. For most students, it is not knowing information in front of their peers that is the most frightening. Remember, if you do not know an answer when questioned in class just say so. Do not delay time or attempt to creatively make something up as doing so will either prompt more questions or unintentionally make a much grander statement of your lack of knowledge. Try not to soil yourself, vomit, or pass out. Know that there are many other classmates that are incredibly thankful you were the "chosen one" as they had no clue of the answer either. For those students who are asked a question and answer correctly, congratulations! However, understand that we tend to ask questions until the endpoint of the students' knowledge is reached. This creates an uncomfortable paradox. If the answer is unknown, the student may be embarrassed in front of their peers, possibly limited on their patient care responsibilities, and ultimately, they will have more questions directed their way. If the student answers correctly, they will most certainly have more questions directed their way. However, they will be trusted with more advanced patient care and the nature of future questions will be different.

---

[4] Karan. Medical students need to be quizzed, but 'pimping' isn't effective. Statnews.com. Published 2017 February 3.
https://www.statnews.com/2017/02/03/medical-students-pimping-testing-knowledge/

The method by which attendings ask questions really is person specific. We all tend to forget that this is your first time in class discussing this subject, or your first rotation with us. We will have had similar experiences with previous students; thus, we may not be as empathetic as we could be. Remember, if your professor or attending is a good-natured person, they most likely did not mean to be cruel. The attending was just progressing through the subject matter and not focusing on your specific sensitivities. Remind yourself to learn from these experiences, and not to dwell in your emotional response to them. If you begin to cry yourself to sleep every time you feel any aspect of negativity, you may as well purchase a waterproof pillow (or try a different career path). Make a concerted effort to adopt the positive teaching approaches taken by the attendings you most admire and to not repeat the negative approaches. Too many students that have undergone a tough educational journey tend to mimic that poor behavior as they advance through the hierarchy. Treating people well through a supportive paradigm while setting high expectations for them tends to be much more productive than a negative based approach.

Being Sent Home

Medical school attracts highly competitive, intelligent, goal-oriented and hardworking individuals. I have been amazed many times by students' dedication, whether it be an 18-hour study day, after hours research project, volunteerism, or those who refuse to go home before completing patient care tasks after their on-call shift ends. As a student/resident, your patient care responsibilities will grow as you advance through the curriculum. It will be tougher to leave the clinic early as your growing expertise will cause you to serve as the director of your team. A smiling hard-working medical student or resident is one of the best gifts any team can receive. However, when your attending sends you home it is important that you listen and GO HOME. There are times for martyrdom, but this is not one of them. If the team has finished its work list and you are dismissed, GO HOME. Sitting in the hospital with the folks who "have" to be there serves no purpose. You will have the rest of your life to heal the infirmed and cure all kinds of pathologies. Take the time you have been given and spend it with your family and/or friends.

On the other hand, asking to be dismissed to go home early is frowned upon and will not earn you points with your team. This is especially true if you are new to the team. For big family occasions, like your wedding or the birth of your child, ask for the time off at the beginning of your rotation. A sentinel family event that suddenly occurs on a day when you are tired will beg legitimacy. Cirque du Soleil does not count as a viable occasion to ask for early dismissal, so don't even think about buying those amazing tickets on Craig's List.

Medical School Changes You

I have yet to meet a person who has completed their training who is not different from who they were before entering the profession. Of course, you will be more learned and have a myriad of experiences that will render you full of information and hopefully some wisdom. That is not what I am talking about. I am talking about the fact that the majority of folks who enter the medical field are high achievers and work hard. They have spent hundreds to thousands of hours preparing for didactics, board exams, and patient care. They have worked weekends, late into the night and forgone sleep. This may sound miserable especially when stated like this. The transition that we all go through with each year of training is amazing. The amount of information we learn and the responsibilities we slowly become comfortable with are unique and special. In my opinion, entering the field of medicine allows us to really live. This is because it is impossible to be a passive bystander of life and active engagement on all levels of humanity is the basic tenant of medicine. That being said we change during the process. A cultural norm within medicine is the constant feedback we all receive whether presenting, making a diagnosis or deliberating a treatment plan. This active feedback is important to us learning from each and every experience, peoples' lives depend on it. This constant feedback does not always feel good. Whether it is delivered in a gentle or not so gentle manner the fact still exists that someone is commenting on work we have done or are doing. Think about the fact that individuals in healthcare work hard and most likely are doing their best. Now add a bit of fatigue and seven years of the monotony to the mix. For those who like equations think of it like this: (high achievers + hard work + fatigue + constant feedback) x at least 7 years = change. Most folks I know become more assertive. This is not a problem if you were shy and soft spoken, it may actually be helpful. However, if you were already outspoken when entering medicine, you may now border on aggressive. I tease one of my closest friends from medical school as I had not ever heard her speak during didactics (years 1 and 2). Though I thought she was mute, she was actually shy and soft spoken. Today she is a pediatrician and I can tell you that I feel bad for anyone who crosses her. She is still gentle in her approach but will not back down from anyone. Today, she is much more likely to tell you what she is thinking than she was when I met her. The importance of this lesson is that it allows us to be somewhat introspective. Pay attention to how we react to the world around us. The world does not know, nor does it care of your sacrifices and it should not be the recipient of your accumulated wrath. We need to protect ourselves from the process, yet allow it to help us become confident enough to govern care in dire situations. By being aware of the process my hope is that you are able to become the person you wish to be both personally and professionally, while not straying too far from your core.

FINANCIAL ADVICE FOR MEDICAL STUDENTS & PROFESSIONALS

Why Money Matters

Discussing your finances with others can be uncomfortable. Talking about finances with medical students or other healthcare professional students (i.e. pharmacists, dentists, optometrists, physician assistants (PAs) and nurses) can be outright scary or even worse—depressing. The topic of money has long been taboo in our society. Personally, my parents were silent, even secretive, when it came to the topic of money; it was something that was not to be talked about. Thus, I never really knew how much my father earned or what our family financial situation was. I remember my childhood friends also being in a similar position as they too never knew how much their parents made let alone any basic knowledge about money.

I grew up extremely poor on Long Island, NY. Neither of my parents graduated high school and we seemed to be always scraping by with my mom sometimes needing to borrow money from me to buy milk. Experiencing poverty served as motivation for me to want to learn more about money and how it worked. As stated in The Millionaire Next Door you will discover that most millionaires did not receive their fortune through inheritance but rather worked hard and earned their wealth. In addition, most of these wealthy Americans are 1st generation millionaires with many of them being immigrants. Thus, one can always hope.

As a 7th grader I purchased two paper routes. The first route was to be delivered in the morning before school and the second was to be delivered after school. I remember as a kid it was hard getting up an hour earlier than everyone else in order to deliver papers. It was even harder work when it was raining, not to mention the dark and cold of winter mornings. It took a lot of discipline to deliver my second route after school when I was tired and many of my friends were out playing. The paper routes did, however, force me to learn how to balance a budget, keep my books, and save money. This basic knowledge and discipline as related to money that I learned as a child has aided me throughout my life and has served as motivation to continually expand my financial knowledge.

Today I am in control of my money and my financial future is bright. It is my goal to help inform you and to turn ignorance into information. By having the ability and discipline to gain entry to college and into a healthcare profession training school, you can most certainly become proficient in the ways of finance. Too frequently, I hear that physicians, pharmacists, dentists, PA's, optometrists and nurses are in financial peril. I believe all medical professionals should have some basic understanding on how to manage money. Unfortunately, this topic is not taught in high school, nor is it covered in college. It is certainly not commonly addressed in medical school, and it is no secret that our profession is terrible with money. Although we rank at near the top of the list for annual income earned nationally,[5] we do not hold that position when it comes to overall net worth.[6] Many healthcare professionals are mission-driven and thus, have chosen a career that provides care for those who are in need. Still, it should not be that our healthcare providers are living paycheck-to-paycheck. Money matters may be the last thing on a physician's mind since our daily business is to concentrate on improving the lives of others. However, this does not mean we should remain ignorant of issues concerning our finances.

---

[5] US News & World Report. Best Paying Jobs. USNEWS.com. Published January 2019. https://money.usnews.com/careers/best-jobs/rankings/best-paying-jobs
[6] Rege, A. 58% of Physicians Have a Net Worth of Less Than $1M: 4 takeaways. Becker's Hospital Review. Published 2018 May 14. https://www.beckershospitalreview.com/hospital-physician-relationships/58-of-physicians-have-a-net-worth-of-less-than-1m-4-takeaways.html

Consider that healthcare professionals work harder than most Americans. Physicians work longer hours than the average American. Doctors work an average 59.6 hours per week as opposed to 44 hours per week for other professions.[7] [8] Physicians also incur much more debt than most Americans and enter the work force later than most Americans do, thereby delaying our ability to save for retirement. Physicians don't start earning a real meaningful salary until the age of 30, and some later than that depending on their specialty and time spent in residency. That equates to being behind our college classmates by 8-10 years in salary generation and retirement saving potential. When the time finally comes to start earning a salary, we must negotiate past more financial obstacles than many others. These include navigating how to pay off a mountain of debt and complying with a progressive tax code targeting high income earners. Many physicians are, in fact, not rich, according to Thomas Stanley author of the Millionaire Next Door and James M. Dahle, M.D, author of The White Coat Investor. In fact, teachers have a higher chance of becoming a millionaire according to Chris Hogan author of Everyday Millionaires. Physicians do not even make the top 3 professions likely to become millionaires despite their high yearly salary.

At a time when 44% of physicians are reporting some kind of burnout and a depression rate of 15%,[9] it is even more critical that we are in a position to be able to negotiate for a fair salary that

[7] Ward, M. A brief history of the 8-hour workday, which changed how Americans work. CNBC.com. Published 2017 May 3. https://www.cnbc.com/2017/05/03/how-the-8-hour-workday-changed-how-americans-work.html
[8] Best Medical Degrees. The Deceptive Salary of Doctors. Bestmedicaldegrees.com. https://www.bestmedicaldegrees.com/salary-of-doctors/
[9] Berg, S. Physician burnout: Which medical specialties feel the most stress. AMA.Org. Published 2019 January 24. https://www.ama-assn.org/practice-management/physician-health/physician-burnout-which-medical-specialties-feel-most-stress

does not require us to work 80-100 hours per week. Our work (and the ever-present reminder of our looming educational debt burden) is often an impediment to having good work/life balance. Take a moment to reflect on how hard you have worked and the time it took you to gain your current expertise. You completed college (most likely at the top of your class). You decided to continue your education with four more years of medical school and three to seven more years of residency (depending on your specialty). You have most likely given up your evenings and weekends for academic pursuits, rather than spending them with friends and family. Taking the appropriate prerequisites and applying to medical school can add at least two more years to the educational process. You have dedicated many years to educating yourself so that you might aid and heal others. It truly is an amazing achievement and a life sacrifice. You have earned the right to balanced life. Understanding your finances, managing your debt, and negotiating favorable salaries and work expectations will help you achieve this.

Are You Worth Your Salary?

The truth is that physician salaries in America need to be higher for many reasons. In fact, not until recently have primary care physicians seen an increase in salary. For many years there has been little to no growth. Why should American physician salaries be high?

Our medical school debt is much higher than that of Europeans. Medical school debt in Europe can average between no indebtedness to $90,000 depending on where training occurs.[10] The Average indebtedness from a public U.S medical school in 2018 was $243,902 and $322,767 for private medical schools,

---

[10] Zavlin D, Jubbal KT, Noé JG, Gansbacher B. A comparison of medical education in Germany and the United States: from applying to medical school to the beginnings of residency. *Ger Med Sci.* 2017;15:Doc15. Published 2017 Sep 25. doi:10.3205/000256

according to the AAMC.org.[11] To put this in perspective, the average undergraduate student loan debt was $29,000.[12] Not to mention that medical school tuition continues to increase, both for private and public schools. A continual 2.9% - 3.6% increase has been occurring for years according to the American Association of Medical Colleges.[13]

We work much harder/longer hours than our European counterparts.[14] European physicians work on average 37-48 hours per week depending on if you live in Denmark or Italy respectively. Take a closer look at a physician's salary and calculate how much we earn per hour; it can be quite educational. When I was in residency from 2003 to 2006, I was earning $42K per year. Working on average 80 hours per week meant that my average hourly rate was $10.50 per hour. My medical assistant with a certification or associate degree essentially made more than I did. Keep in mind, while physicians are in residency training, undergraduate and medical school loans continue to earn interest, even on loans that are in deferment. The residency salary is enough for physicians to live off, but its limitations make loan repayment extremely difficult.

Now, let us jump ahead to an attending's salary. If, for example I make $186,000 per year. You might think that's outstanding. It's true, it's not a bad salary. However, when broken down it begins to illustrate the hourly wage is not as high as you might think. Take $186,000 and divide it by 52 weeks and then divide by 40 hours per week and you come up with $90/hour. Not bad, right? No

---

[11] Budd, K. 7 ways to reduce medical school debt. AAMC.org. Published 2018 October 9. https://www.aamc.org/news-insights/7-ways-reduce-medical-school-debt

[12] CollegeBoard. Trends in Student Aid 2019, Cumulative Debt: Bachelor's Degree Recipients. CollegeBoard.com. Published 2019 November. https://research.collegeboard.org/pdf/2019-trendsinsa-fig14.pdf

[13] AAMC. Tuition and Student Fees Reports. AAMC.org. Published 2019 October. https://www.aamc.org/data/tuitionandstudentfees/

[14] It is very hard to gather data on this subject but data from 2014 indicates the number of hours depends on each country with countries like Denmark physicians working 37 hours per week and other countries such as Austria, Italy and Portugal have work limitations of 48 hours.

physician works 40 hours, and as the number of hours increases so the hourly wage decreases. So, if we use the same formula, but increase the work time to 80 hours per week, attending physicians only make about $45 per hour. (This, however, does not yet account for taxes, which we will discuss later.)

Our post graduate training results in a delayed ability to build wealth. Many of our collegiate buddies obtained a job after graduating, they begin paying off debt and start to accumulate wealth. However, when future doctors leave college, they enroll in an additional 7-12 years of training, delaying their ability to earn an income, pay off student loans, and contribute to savings. A 22 year-old recent college graduate can start to save for retirement by contributing $200 each month to their 401K plan. If they continue this habit until the age of 65, assuming annual rate of return of 10%, this person would retire with a nest egg of $1,575,986. Using the same parameters for calculating returns, the residency trained physician starting to save for retirement at age 32 has 10 less years to save. This physician's nest egg would only reach $591,389 by the age of 65 (see figure 1). It is a big deal to lose that much time and start so late. Starting late to save for retirement always means you'll have to save more from your monthly income to catch up, and potentially retire later in life.

Figure 1: Balance of 401k Savings at Retirement

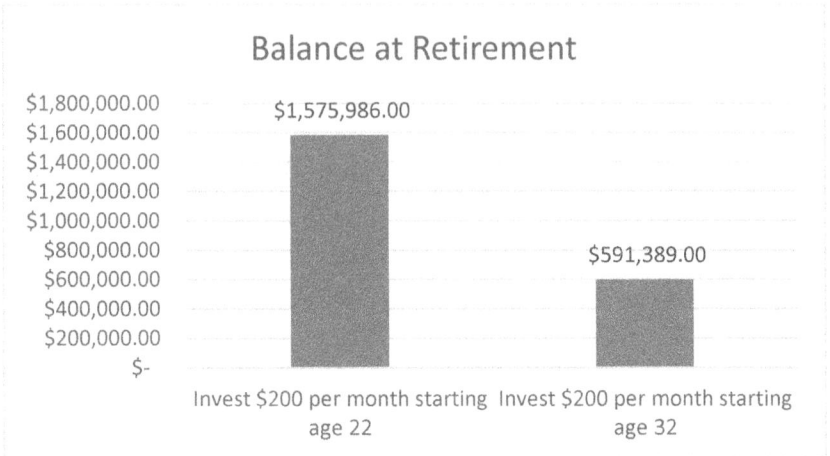

Balance at Retirement

Invest $200 per month starting age 22: $1,575,986.00

Invest $200 per month starting age 32: $591,389.00

In America, the higher your gross income, the more you pay in annual taxes. You need to know that taxes will have the biggest impact on your financial situation. They will negatively affect your bottom line -more than your mortgage, student loans and credit cards. Our country uses a progressive tax code both federally and on the state level. This means that the more you work, the more you make, the more you will have to pay. Many physicians will pay up to 30-50% of their income in taxes per year.

So, are physicians really worth their salaries? They incur massive amounts of debt to become doctors. They work longer and harder than the average 40-hour work week. Their ability to save and build wealth is delayed by roughly a decade as they pursue medical training. And, a significant portion of their income is automatically reserved for taxes. When you factor all of this in, doctors are not banking as much as it would seem.

Physicians and Money

I tend to ask a lot of questions. This accomplishes two things: first, it really embarrasses my wife; secondly, it serves as a vehicle for discovering what others are doing with their money. I usually approach accomplished physicians (who by my calculations should be extremely wealthy) whom are likely able to give me sound financial advice. I approach specialists (surgeons, gastroenterologists and dermatologists, etc.) to learn what they are doing with their earnings. These specialties usually rank among the highest paid within our profession. I thought that these highly-paid individuals would have accumulated enough wealth to retire early. What I discovered was astounding—most of my colleagues where not rich at all. Yes, they had very high salaries; but, they also had beautiful luxury cars, very large houses, and essentially, I found that they lived above their means. However, they did not have much put away for retirement.

I was completely shocked. This really interested me; thus, I leaned in to learn more. A larger number of these specialist physicians were divorced (22% for primary care and 33% for specialists). I will not delve into the reason that so many providers are divorced, but work hours are often a factor. These divorces add an additional financial strain to an already highly taxed income. Opening a private clinical practice also seems to account for many physicians' financial woes. We spend our time learning medicine and think that it translates into a successful business model—for many it does not. Practicing physicians do not have time, nor have most doctors taken the time to learn the financial side of running a practice. Being a good doctor and being a good businessperson are two distinct skill sets. As my brother-in-law tells me, "physicians have a big shovel" and can dig their way out of most financial crisis. This means our income is large enough that recovering from a financial mistake or investment is usually shorter and less painful than for many others. So, there is hope for us. However, with a lack of financial discipline, many in our profession continue to make the same mistakes. Other financial mistakes that physicians make include purchasing high cost items such as houses, boats, cars and time shares too soon after residency. Think about it, there is really little benefit on saving a few dollars at the grocery store with your coupons if you're going to buy a time share for $40,000 and only use it once per year.

The Cost of Becoming a Physician

Getting an advanced medical degree can be extremely expensive. The price of medical school and the enormous debt we physicians and other medical professionals find ourselves in after residency and training is mind boggling. Gone are the days of paying off your medical school loans five years out of residency. In the 1980's and 1990's, physicians would leave school with a manageable amount of debt which translated into their ability to pay off their loans quickly. Data from AMSA.org indicates the average tuition for public medical school at that time was $2,781 per year and $8,962 per year for private.[15] After factoring in for cost of living, you might be looking at a total medical education debt burden of $40,000 for public institutions and $70,000 for private schools. The average physician salary in 1982 was $125,500, which allowed them to have an easier time paying off their loans.[16] I sometimes hear seasoned physicians giving new graduates an ear full for the "indentured servitude" they are about to enter. How much has really changed over time? Physician salaries have not kept up proportionally with medical school debt. 35 years ago, a family medicine doctor might leave residency with $70,000 of medical school loans from private medical school with a starting salary of $125,000. This translates to a salary to debt ratio of 1.8. Today many newly minted attendings leave residency with $322,000 of private medical school loans and a starting salary of $223,000. That translates to a salary to debt ratio of 0.69. (See figure 2.) In this example, the salary has increased by 78%, but the student loans have increased by 360%. The situation can be even more unsettling if the physician owes money from their undergraduate studies.

---

[15] American Medical Student Association. Medical School Tuition Frequently Asked Questions. AMSA.org. https://www.amsa.org/advocacy/action-committees/twp/tuition-faq/

[16] Pope, GC and Schneider, JE. Data Watch: Trends in physician income. HealthAffairs.Org. https://www.healthaffairs.org/doi/pdf/10.1377/hlthaff.11.1.181

Figure 2. Physician Salary to Debt Ratio

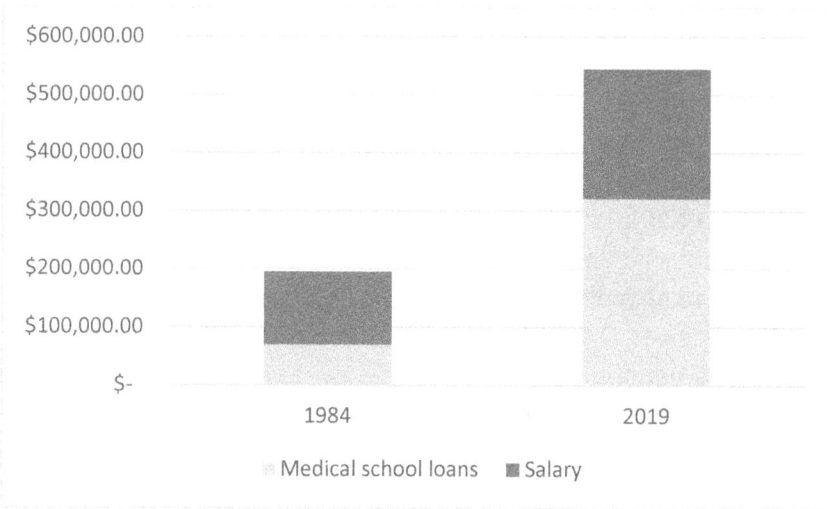

Private schools are costlier than state schools and osteopathic schools are usually more costly than allopathic schools.

Figure 3. Average medical tuition cost in 2018-2019[17]

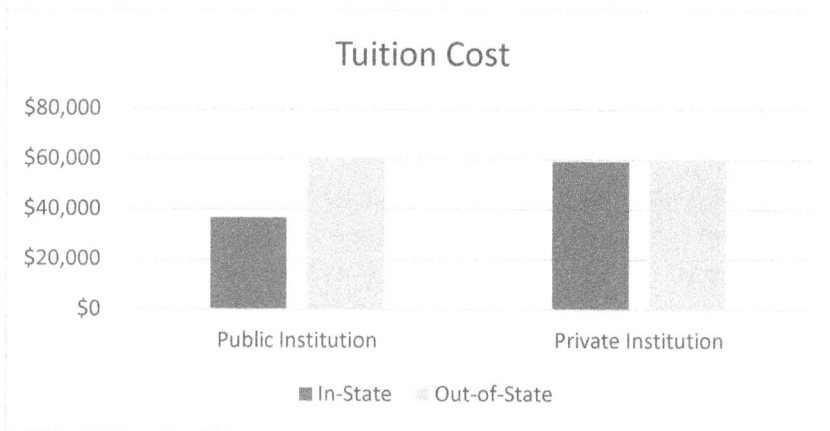

[17] AAMC. Tuition and Student Fees Reports. AAMC.org. Published 2019 October. https://www.aamc.org/data/tuitionandstudentfees/

Physician Debt

I am sure you have heard that debt is bad and should be avoided at all costs. Dave Ramsey has entire books on how to minimize and eliminate your debt. (I recommend reading any/all of his books.) In the case of medical professionals, debt that most of us cannot avoid. The cost of education, especially medical education, is so high that it has outpaced inflation and earnings and having school debt is commonly considered a part of the process. I sometimes ask medical students how high their debt load is. They typically answer: "I don't know;" "It's too depressing for me to look;" or "There's nothing I can do about it now".

The interest rates today are also quite high, varying between 6.25 - 7%.[18] In 2010, the federal government took control of all student loans. The loans are now provided directly from the Department of Education to students. Federal education loans are unsecured loans with no collateral. Higher interest rates are expected in part because the default rate and thus risk to the institution (the government) is higher. A home mortgage has a lower interest rate. If you fail to pay, the bank will repossess your home and sell the house to recoup the loss. If you do not pay your student loans, they do not come to your home and extract the education from your brain. The government has to absorb that cost.

A student loan debt burden is typically more than the amount of the loan initially borrowed. These loans also accrue interest until they are paid off. This includes the time during medical school (4 years) and residency (3-7 years) while the loans are in deferment. Let's consider an OB/GYN resident who graduates from a private medical school with $400,000 in school loans at a 6% interest rate. The OB/GYN residency lasts 4 years; and interest accrues each year. After 4 years, not including minimal payments, they would owe $504,990. That's an increase of more than $100,000! While

---

[18] Nykiel, T. What Is the Average Medical School Debt? Nerdwallet.com. Published 2019 December 17. https://www.nerdwallet.com/blog/loans/student-loans/average-medical-school-debt/

it is a good idea to pay toward your loans during residency, the average resident salary of $59,300 yearly makes it hard to put a substantial dent in any principle.[19] You would be lucky to pay down ¼ of the interest ($500/month of the total interest of $2,000/month) monthly. Remember while in residency you also need to pay for rent/mortgage, transportation, insurance, food, utilities and clothes. $59K does not get you very far. Imagine trying to get by on $59K per year with a spouse and 2 kids at home. Some residents may try to pay as little as they can in an income-based payment plan. These plans are functional in the short term, but increase the problem in the long term as the interest on their loans continues to accrue.

Figure 4. Average Amount of Debt for the Class of 2018[20]

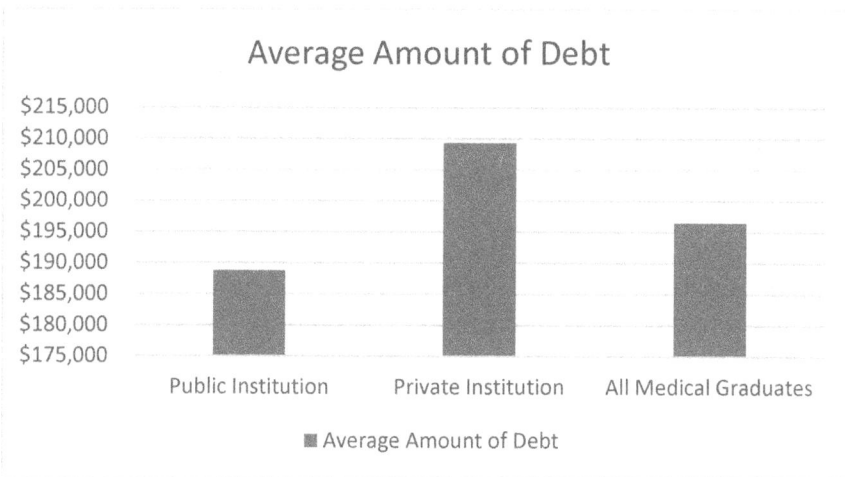

Average Amount of Debt

---

[19] The Do Staff. What residents are getting paid in 2019. TheDo.Osteopathic.Org. Published 2018 July 23. https://thedo.osteopathic.org/2018/07/what-residents-are-getting-paid-in-2018/

[20] AAMC Financial Information, Service, Resources and Tools. Medical student education: Debt, costs and loan repayment fact card 2018 (pdf). AAMC.Org. Published 2018. https://store.aamc.org/medical-student-education-debt-costs-and-loan-repayment-fact-card-2018-pdf.html

53

Taxes

I currently serve as the faculty representative to the Business of Medicine Club for the university at which I teach. Each year I have the opportunity to give a short one-hour lecture on personal finance. Annually, I ask those in the audience (typically 1st and 2nd year medical students) what they believe will be there largest debt/bill after medical school. I usually give them choices such as the mortgage, medical school loans, utilities, car payment and credit cards. As I have stated prior, it is none of those items. It is TAXES.

Physicians are typically in the top 5% income earners. Specialists often fall into the top 1-2%. Many new attending physicians are shocked after viewing their 1st real physician paycheck. As after a decade of training (and tangential building of debt), they wait in happy anticipation for their "big" paycheck hoping it will solve their financial woes. Reality sets in when they take a glimpse at their net pay. The attending sits and stares at their paycheck in disbelief as up to 40% of their predicted take home funds may be missing.

Many physicians may have prematurely performed what I call "physician math", and are ill-prepared for this new financial reality. Physician Math calculations tend to go like this: *I earned $50K per year as a resident and took home $1,500 every 2 weeks. So, now that I'm an attending OB/GYN physician with an annual salary of $300,000, I should expect my net pay to increase six-fold just like my annual pay. This means I should get $9,000 every 2 weeks.* They are disappointed when their real net pay is only about $6,600 and, often, they do not understand what caused the discrepancy. This phenomenon is called the progressive tax code. If you earn more than $130k per year (that will be all of you) you will be enrolled in the Alternative Minimal Tax program (AMT). It is an extremely complicated federal tax program, but essentially it means that you will be taxed at a higher rate than other citizens who earn less in wages. Many of you may now owe income taxes come April. The change in your tax rate is usually not apparent during the 1st year post residency because you would only have received a high salary for about five months. The next tax year is when the real awakening occurs. After making a full attending salary for one year (January – December) the following April can be a big shocker. Many physicians can owe as much as $20-$50k. A very large sum to come up with if you are not prepared. More financially astute physicians will save all year in anticipation of paying taxes; or they will pay extra on a quarterly basis to ease the pain come tax time.

OK. Enough bad news. How can I change my financial stars?

A Cautionary Tale (My Story)

It was February 2008. Standing in my kitchen after a long day's work as an active Air Force Family Medicine physician, I heard my wife begin to cry. I initially thought she was upset with my long hours and my inability to spend quality time with my new family. At that point, we had 2 boys under the age of 2. I thought to myself, "surely, she must understand," as she was working as a part-time pediatric hospitalist. Then she said "I can't take it anymore. All we do is work. Most of the money goes elsewhere. When do we get to enjoy the benefits of our labor?" I knew money was tight but did not know just how tight. Our arrangement was that I would pay the mortgage from my earnings and she would take care of the rest of the bills. At that time we lived in Arizona and our mortgage was $4,600 per month (which took up my entire monthly military salary). School loan payments for both of us were $1,500 per month, our car payments were $800 per month, plus we spent over $1,500 monthly for various other bills such as credit cards, utilities, food, childcare and essentials. My military salary and my wife's part-time pediatrician salary was simply not enough. We did exactly what I warned you all about. We were foolish after residency and bought too much house. We got caught up in the housing bubble and purchased our house for $644,000 in 2006. We thought we could afford it. We were physicians now and thought things would work themselves out. As previously stated, my mortgage was

$4,600 per month at a 7% interest rate. Each month $500 went to the principle and $4,100 went to interest, taxes and insurance. The main problem was we did not have a plan to attack our debt. When I say plan, I really mean a BUDGET. We did not know the sum of our expenses. I did not even know my wife's take-home pay. We were financially disorganized. We were not communicating and it was starting to affect our marriage.

So, what did we do? Well, I was unexpectedly deployed to Iraq. Oddly enough, I had significant down time abroad and while there I decided to come up with a plan to get our family out of this financial quagmire. Luckily, I came upon a financial course being offered at the base chapel in Balad, Iraq. It was called Financial Peace University. A 13-week personal finance course offered by Dave Ramsey. Can you believe it? In a war zone, I was learning personal finance. Dave Ramsey is a patriot and donated his course to all active duty servicemen on deployment. In those 13 weeks, the forty or so attendants dropped 1.2 million in debt. Those 13 weeks changed my life. What I learned allowed me to help steer our family towards eventually dumping an enormous amount of debt. The time spent understanding finances also motivated me to the proactive management of our finances. I read *The Millionaire Next Door*, *The Richest Man in Babylon* and *The Truth About Money*. I drew up a budget, tightened our purse strings, and when I got home things began to change. Initially it was tough getting my wife on board as she thought I wanted us to live like college students. In truth, I did want to severely scale back our spending and after multiple energetic conversations we compromised. My wife started to buy into the process and within 4 and ½ years our net worth changed from minus $208,000 to positive 1 million. I could not believe it. We were not surgeons nor were we highly paid specialists. We were two primary care physicians earning relatively low physician salaries—mine, an Air Force salary, and my wife's, that of a part-time pediatric hospitalist. What is important to realize is that it is not the amount of money you gross, nor is it the amount of money you net that plays the critical role. It is the amount of money that you KEEP that matters.

How did our transition occur? It all started with paying off our car debt. YES. Paying off the cars. Next, I learned fiscal discipline for the second time in my life (remember the paper route?). Third, my wife got on board and became an active participant and driver of the plan. Before I knew It, I had money in the bank and could keep a few of my paychecks. Credit card balances disappeared. An emergency fund was created and saving for our retirement took priority. As you look toward your financial future as a physician, remember NOT to start as I did. Rather, do some planning now to set yourself up for greater financial success.

8 Steps for Financial Planning

Step 1: Understand your financial situation

If you are a 2nd year medical student and do not know how much you owe in loans or do not know the interest rate on said loans, learn it now. What are the terms of your loans, how long will it take for you to pay them off? How much do you owe on credit cards and/or auto loans?

While on a recent deployment to Qatar, I was talking with one of my flight surgery colleagues about finance. He was one year out of internship and working in flight medicine but still hoping to get a residency in dermatology. I told him I was writing this chapter regarding finances. He became very interested in the topic and wanted to learn more. I gave him a few of the books that I had read, and he started attending some financial forums the base provided. Initially, he shared with me that he owed $383,000 in medical school loans. When he looked up his loans to show me later, we discovered that he actually owed $424,000. He had forgotten about the interest.

Remember as a medical student, intern or newly graduated resident you need to live below your means to achieve financial success. Graduating residency does not mean you should immediately buy a new car, buy a large dream house, and take lavish vacations. This will happen in due time, believe me. Yes, I am suggesting that you prolong your gratification once more. This may be especially tough on your spouse or significant other if they have different expectations, so engage in this journey together. The compromise my wife and I made was quite simple. No, we would not live like residents again. What we did is live somewhere in between our resident salary and attending salary. That plan was extremely effective in leaving more money at the end of the month to pay down debt and allow us to save. I can't tell you the joy, satisfaction and security we felt having $20K in the bank in case of an emergency. The anxiety that lived in our chests was fading and we were starting to make active life decisions rather than let life make the decisions for us.

Step 2: Create a budget and calculate your net worth (write or type it out)

This will serve as the foundation of your plan and the source of your personal financial knowledge. You need to know how much money is coming in and how much is going out each month. In the beginning, this budget should be completed monthly. It's so easy these days using an excel spreadsheet and should only take 30-40 minutes once your initial budget is constructed. I know many of you do not have a steady stream of income and you may think writing a budget is absurd but knowing your financial reality will put you on a tract to success. Creating a budget will also curb your spending by providing a feedback loop to the decisions you make and how they affect you financially. This should help you develop the lifelong habit of living below your means. It will allow you to realize how fast your money goes and exactly where you spend most of your resources. You can find numerous budget forms online. (Evaluate the resources at daveramsey.com!) If you are intimidated by too many columns and calculations, write out a simple budget first. After you get used to the process you can move onto a more advanced version. Get your partner involved and include your kids in what you learn. Bounce ideas back and forth between each other. It truly can be a fun process.

Step 3: Get rid of the car payment

Annually, at the beginning of each medical school year I watch in shock as new 1st year med students arrive on campus in their new cars. The same trend occurred in my last year of residency as one of my fellow residents purchased a new Lexus at a cost of $60,000. If the car is not paid for in full it will require a steep monthly payment. I typically hear a student saying, "I'm from California and my parents wanted to make sure I had a reliable car". I personally drive a 2008 Camry which has never broken down and has no car payment, and I'm a millionaire. I can also say, it's reliable. Getting rid of the car payment, saving on the car insurance and registration will ultimately free up a bunch of money to pay down general debt or better off reduce the amount of student debt you are about to take out. If you avoid purchasing a new car, the amount of savings from this step alone will yield significant monetary benefit in the coming years due to the reduction in compound interest. The $10,000 auto loan you take out today will not be $10,000 when you pay it back. After 20 years at 7% interest, it will amount to over $18,000. Hence, it is best to reduce the amount of loans you take out initially. Remember interest starts accruing immediately. This means that, yes, interest will accumulate while you are in medical school.

While on deployment in Iraq I had a roommate, who was determined to buy himself a new BMW once his 6-month tour was over. He was a nurse and a 1st lieutenant making good money. While on deployment we don't have to pay federal taxes and thus he technically got a big raise. He believed he could save up half the price of the car and his car payments on the remaining balance would be $500 per month for 5 years. Of course he did not want to get a basic BMW, but rather he wanted the high-end model. After a few weeks of deployment and many conversations, he agreed to take the same financial course I took. By the time we left Iraq he decided to buy a 3-year-old used BMW for less than ½ the price of the new version and no car payments. He was a changed man.

Step 4: Don't use credit cards

I think most of us know that using credit cards can become habit forming. I liken credit cards and their misuse to gambling. The thrill people get from buying something new is very addicting. If you really have a problem with using plastic, you may need professional help. Please go and get it. The military takes this topic very seriously and offers counseling to those in need to help kick the habit. In place of the credit cards, I would advise using a debit card, or even better, pay with cash. Paying with cash makes the process of buying something more painful for the spender. It requires a taking trip to the ATM where you see your balance drop and then you must physically hand over the cash to the store cashier. For most people, this is not at all thrilling. We all hate receiving a high credit card bill, and having the question if there has been a mistake or if we really spent that much. If this happens to you frequently, you need to make some changes to better understand your spending habits and stay on budget. If you cannot afford to purchase something in the moment, then do not buy it on credit. Think of it this way, if you cannot afford to buy it now, you most likely will not be able to afford the item plus interest at a later date.

Step 5: Don't buy "too much" house

Buying a house is potentially the biggest financial decision you will make and should not be taken lightly. I made the mistake of buying too much house, too soon and paid for it (literally and figuratively) for many years post the purchase. If you are to buy a house please look at the amortization schedule to understand just how much of your monthly payment will go to interest and principle over time. This will also help you delineate how much you are paying towards PMI (private mortgage insurance) and property taxes.

I wish someone would have told me to do this the first time I bought a house. The first 5-7 years of your 30-year mortgage payments will hardly put a dent in your principle, most of the money goes toward interest. A 15-year mortgage, however, saves you on interest and time. These loans typically offer a lower interest rate and you will be able to pay down your principle more quickly, though the principle payment will be higher. I would also advise putting down at least 20% on your house to avoid PMI. PMI can sometimes cost you $200 per month and provides nothing for you. It is the bank's insurance you will not default on the loan. Individuals with less than 20% stake in their homes are more apt to leaving their mortgage unpaid. Another option that many physicians consider getting is the "Doctors Loan", which only requires a 3% down payment. There are various organizations that will offer you this. I would not recommend taking this type of approach to purchasing a house. Having less than a 20% down payment is an indicator that you are buying too much house.

Remember, big houses need to be furnished, repaired, cooled and heated. They also need to be covered by insurance. All of this always costs more than you anticipate. Depending on where you settle, your home may need landscaping and yard care. I know, you are the do-it-yourself type and you want to mow your own lawn. However, when you consider that working 1½ to 2 times longer than most Americans does not leave much time at the end of the day to complete your charts, spend time with the family, exercise and eat, you will realize that yardwork becomes a lower priority. When you factor in the time it takes to complete yard work and the time value of money, you will most likely conclude that it is better to pay someone else to do it. Is your partner a stay-at-home partner or one who works? I ask because big houses need to be cleaned, a task that can take many hours. If you have a stay-at-home spouse, they may agree to clean the house when not caring for the children and running errands. Being a stay-at-home parent is the toughest job in existence, and there is often no free time to clean. As a physician, you certainly will not want to start house cleaning after a 14-16-hour clinical day. This usually means that you will need a house cleaner, which can cost about $100-$150 every two weeks for a large house. This is an additional cost and adds to your expenses. Thus, buying a house that is "just big enough" is a much better option than buying too much house. Frequently this means your home will cost less, meaning a smaller monthly payment. Plus, a smaller yard, and smaller area to clean can decrease (or eliminate) the costs for the additional services.

Step 6: Start saving for retirement ASAP

I know this goes against many financial gurus who state you need to pay off all debt before contributing to retirement, but that's for the average college grad with 30k in debt. Physicians laugh at such a minuscule number. Many of my colleagues at the age of 50 are still paying off their medical school loans. At 50 years of age it is too late to start saving for retirement. At that point, you have lost the time value of money and power of accrued interest. Just like interest on your student loans accrues to your detriment, interest on your investments accrues to your benefit. Therefore, you should start early and be a consistent contributor. I put the maximum amount allowable into my retirement savings and so does my wife. It comes directly out of my paycheck every two weeks; and after a while, it is not even money that I miss. My budget does not consider that money as earned income because it is taken from my gross wages rather than my net pay. Your retirement savings contributions also qualify as a tax break, lowering your overall tax bill at the end of the year (something you will desperately need). If you are lucky enough to have a 401K or 403B, maximize them.

Step 7: Have someone else pay off your loans

This is a big topic and one which needs to be looked at carefully. First, I would like to say most physicians do not stay employed at their initial post-residency job for very long. Physicians tend to change jobs every 3-5 years. Around 50% of physicians leave the profession after five years. When transitioning jobs, remember to negotiate for someone to cover your *tail coverage* (that's a topic for another time). This is beneficial for many reasons. I mentioned that you should start saving for retirement before paying off your student loans. Did you know that many employers will pay down your loan debts for you? Sign-on bonuses and loan forgiveness programs can be negotiated in your contract. These help tremendously toward alleviating the financial burden of student debt. Also of note, utilizing these programs will not decrease your salary. It is major plus, but can come with some obligations. Sign-on bonuses are typically taxed at a higher rate.

There are various programs to consider which will help with your loan indebtedness. One that I am fairly familiar with is the Health Professions Scholarship Program, sponsored by the U.S. military. The Army, Navy, Air Force and Public Health service provide students with a full scholarship to medical school with the addition of books, health care and a little over $2,000 per month stipend. These scholarships are in my opinion one of the best avenues available to advancing your financial stability. Imagine leaving medical school with no debt. Similar programs offer three and four-year scholarships for continuing medical students, and the Navy and Army offer a $20K sign-on bonus to participants. (The Air Force does not provide a sign-on bonus.) This program requires a three to four-year military commitment after residency, so weigh out the pros and cons of this requirement before enrolling in the program.

The Reserve/National Guard also has programs to assist in debt forgiveness if you do not sign up for service before or during medical school. These programs are available to you during residency and they can boost your resident salary considerably. Similarly, these require a service commitment of several years as a reservist. After my active duty military commitment (HPSP scholarship payback) I signed with the Air Force Reserve and received a $75K bonus over three years!

There are also multiple loan repayment programs for those who agree to work in an under-resourced environment.[21] While in some states this would mean practicing in a rural town, this is not

---

[21] Research National Public Health Service Repayment Program, National Institute of Health Repayment Program, Public Service Loan Forgiveness Program (federal loans), and also consider state and local repayment programs.

true everywhere. The goal is to station providers in an area where the provider to patient ratio is skewed to where there are many people with few providers. If you are not interested in practicing in rural Mississippi, do not worry. These areas also exist within most cities.

Step 8: Choose your Residency location carefully

Finding a geographical home and practice is a huge decision, especially if you have a spouse and children to consider. Being near relatives, living in the climate that is right for you, and being happy with your salary and position all come into play when making this decision. A general assumption is that living anywhere near one of the coasts of the United States equals higher housing and living costs. It may also mean lower pay as others want to live there and will work harder for lower wages. The combination of higher living cost and lower salary with an already high education debt burden can make for increased stress, especially in a new marriage. Some folks want to live near NYC, Boston and Washington D.C. in order to enjoy the culture, fine food options and amenities that the location offers. Others want to live near the beaches in Honolulu, Miami and San Diego. The problem is everyone else has the same idea, making positions in these regions highly competitive. The big cities and nice weather attract multitudes of people including other medical professionals. Many of these states have steep progressive state taxes, which will severely bite into your take home pay and hamper your ability to save for retirement.

I have often talked with my wife about moving to California. We frequently go and visit her parents who live in Orange County and after a week of being there, we come home to Arizona and take a deep sigh of relief. We celebrate the freedom of the roads, the open spaces, and the tranquility. Did I mention we also have a lower cost of living? You can live in those highly coveted states if you so choose, but understand how that choice impacts your finances and, ultimately, your quality of life. I have calculated the amount we have saved in state taxes by not living in California. In over 20 years at our current combined salary, we have saved $25-30k per year or $500-600k total. We have chosen instead to put that money toward retirement in an effort to earn the freedom of choice in our later years. The bottom line is living in places like New York or California may seem nice at first, but can potentially make it extremely tough to get ahead financially.

Hume's Helpful Habits

<u>Live below your means</u> – This single piece of advice may be all that you need to win financially. It will also protect you against negative life events such as losing a job or you being out of work due to illness or disability.

<u>Adopt a plan</u> – Start a budget! Calculate your monthly income, and track your net worth and spending habits quarterly.

<u>Don't use credit cards</u> – Use cash instead. If you must use them, pay the entire balance every month – most people don't (not even doctors).

<u>Don't buy a new car</u> – Just because you are a physician doesn't mean you "deserve" a new vehicle. A two-year-old model looks just as new and can save you a bundle. Never have a car payment – This is one of the 1st steps to financial freedom. It frees up cash to pay down debt or invest.

<u>Don't buy "too much" house</u> – Honestly how many square feet do you need? Buying a mansion is just showing off and can severely restrict your ability to save for the future.

<u>Get a 15-year mortgage</u> – Nothing says you must have a 30-year mortgage. Getting the 15-year variety will allow you to get a lower interest rate and save many thousands of dollars in interest.

Start saving for retirement ASAP – As physicians we are behind most others in our age group regarding saving for retirement. Because of our lengthy education, we enter the work force late, and therefore lose precious time investing in our futures. We need to catch up, so start saving immediately.

Have someone else pay off your student loans – As we discussed, many employers will offer this as a benefit. Be sure to bring it up in contract negotiations!

Consider where to live – States on the coasts tend to pay less and have a higher rate for income taxes. If you live in places like NY, NJ, CT, and CA, you may find it hard to get ahead with the high housing prices and steep progressive tax codes.

Continue to educate yourself about finances – Pick up *The White Coat Investor*, *The Millionaire Next Door*, or *Financial Peace*. All these books are must reads.

Start and maintain a nice fat emergency fund – It is not out of the realm of possibility to have $50,000 in the bank. Having an emergency fund will protect you from spiraling after life's bumps, and it allows you to sleep at night.

Book List

The following books are a must read for any medical student or medical professional

1. *The Richest Man in Babylon* – George Samuel Clason
2. *The White Coat Investor* – James M. Dahle, MD
3. *The Truth About Money* – Ric Edelman
4. *Everyday Millionaires* – Chris Hogan
5. *Retire Inspired* – Chris Hogan
6. *Rich Dad, Poor Dad* – Robert T. Kiyosaki
7. *Thou Shall Prosper* – Daniel Lapin
8. *Financial Peace* – Dave Ramsey
9. *Total Money Makeover* – Dave Ramsey
10. *The Millionaire Next Door* – Thomas J. Stanley & William D. Danko
11. *Stop Acting Rich* – Thomas J. Stanley

About the Authors

Alan Schalscha, D.O., M.S., C.P.E. is a family medicine physician and associate professor in Texas. A graduate of UT Austin and Chief Medical Officer of CommUnityCare. He completed his Master of Science at the University of North Texas, and his medical education at Midwestern University (School of Osteopathic Medicine) in Arizona. There is an advancing shortage of physicians both in primary and specialty care. In an effort to demystify the process and increase participation Dr. Schalscha hopes that in writing this book, he can help more students gain an understanding of what medical school and training is really like.

David Hume, D.O. is a family medicine physician and associate professor in Arizona. A graduate of SUNY – Oswego, he earned a cytology certification from the University of Miami school of Medicine in Florida, before befriending Dr. Schalscha while they studied together at Midwestern University. Dr. Hume has served as a medical officer in multiple branches of the armed forces (Air Force, Air Force Reserve, and Army Reserve), and it was during his time of service that he began to learn—and to share with others—tips and strategies for personal finance management.

Appendices
Appendix I
Alan Schalscha, D.O., M.S., CPE

Education

CPE, American Association for Physician Leadership, Tampa, FL	2014
D.O., Midwestern University, Arizona College of Osteopathic Medicine, Glendale, Arizona	2003
M.S., Physiology, The University of North Texas Health Science Center, Ft. Worth, TX	1998
B.A., Biology, The University of Texas, Austin, TX	1995
B.A., Anthropology, The University of Texas, Austin, TX	1992

Postdoctoral Training

Resident; Chief Resident, St. Joseph's Hospital and Medical Center, Phoenix, AZ   2004 – 2006
Internship, University of New Mexico Health Science Center, Albuquerque, NM   2003 - 2004

Licensure
Texas Medical Board
Board Certification/Eligibility

Texas Medical Board	2016 - Present
American Board of Family Medicine	2006 - Present
Arizona Board of Osteopathic Examiners in Medicine and Surgery	2006 – 2016

Academic and Leadership Appointments

Clinical Associate Professor   2016 - Present
Department of Population Health, The University of Texas Dell Medical School, Austin, TX
Interim Chief of Family Medicine   2019 – 01/2020
Department of Population Health, The University of Texas Dell Medical School, Austin, TX
Chief Medical Officer, CommUnityCare Health Centers, Austin, TX
                                                                                       2016 - Present
Clinical Associate Professor   2012 - 2016
AT Still University, Mesa, AZ
Chief Medical Officer, HonorHealth NOAH Clinics, Scottsdale, AZ 2011 - 2016
Course Director and Clinical Associate Professor   2011 - 2012
Clinical Medicine, Midwestern University School of Optometry, Glendale, AZ
Course Director and Clinical Associate Professor   2007 - 2012
Midwestern University School of Medicine, Glendale, AZ

Other Relevant Employment and Clinical Activities

Family Medicine Clinic Coordinator/Director and Physician,   2007 - 2011
Midwestern University Multi-Specialty Clinic, Glendale, AZ
Co-Director, Co-Founder, Humanity Eye and Tissue Bank, Phoenix, AZ
                                                                                           2007 - 2010
Physician, James Dearing, D.O. Family Medicine, Phoenix, AZ   2006 - 2007

Honors and Awards

Travis County Medical Society Humanitarian of the Year Award   2019

Dr. John Burdick Humanitarian Award – Honoring Service to International
Under-resourced   2016

Most Approachable Professor - Student Choice Award   2013
Earnest A. Allaby Award – Honoring: International Medical Outreach
                                                               2012
Professor of the Year Award - Midwestern University, Student Choice Award
                                                               2012
Humanitarian of the Year Award - Arizona Osteopathic Medical Association
                                                               2010
The LittleJohn Award - Midwestern University- Highest Service Award
                                                               2009
Most Caring Professor of the Year - Student Choice Award, Midwestern
University   2009
Nomination - AOA Mentor of the Year - Elected to AOA Hall of Fame
                                                               2008
Top Forty Under 40 – Top Forty Leaders in Arizona Under 40 Years of Age,
                                                               2008
Phoenix Business Journal
Best New Professor – Student Choice Award, Midwestern University   2008
Dr. Lee Parker Davis Humanitarian of the Year Award,   2006
St. Joseph's Hospital & Medical Center

Professional Memberships and Activities with Leadership Positions
TMA/TCMS   2016 - Present
American Medical Association   2003 - Present
American Osteopathic Association   2003 - Present
American Association of Family Physicians   2003 - Present

Educational Activities

Educational Administration and Leadership
Member, Pediatric Chair Search Committee, Dell Medical School   2019
Member, Population Health Chair Search Committee, Dell Medical School
                                                   2019 – Present

Member, LCME Standard 5 Committee, Dell Medical School   2019
Member, Dean's Preceptor Review Advisory Council, Midwestern University
                                                   2010 - 2011

Member, Best Practices Committee, Midwestern University   2008 - 2011

Member, Student Promotions Committee, Midwestern University   2008 - 2010
Chair, MSI Student Liaison Committee, Midwestern University   2008 - 2009
Member, MSI Student Liaison Committee, Midwestern University   2007 - 2009
President, Arizona Chief Resident Consortium   2005 - 2006

Teaching Activities
The University of Texas at Austin

Healthcare Career Development Lecture Series for UT Student Athletes
05/13/2019
University of Texas Athletes Pre-Health Organization

11/13/2019
Primary Care Clerkship Didactics – Hypertension Lecture   08/07/2019
Dell Medical School
Primary Care, Family and Community Medicine Clerkship   2017 - Present
Dell Medical School (various dates)

AT Still University
Introduction to Clinical Medicine, Clinical Associate Professor   2012 - 2016
Department of Family Medicine, 120 students, all of the following were taught
but differed annually based on my availability, Introduction to History and
Physical, SOAP notes, Vitals, Head and Neck, EENT, HEENT Lab, Newborn
Exam, HEENT H&P, Cardiovascular Exam, Respiratory Exam, Heart and Lung
Lab, Abdominal Exam, Well Child/Adolescent Exam, Abdominal Exam, Male
Genitourinary, Musculoskeletal Exam, Neurology Exam,
Musculoskeletal Lab, Pediatrics, Female Genitourinary Exam

Midwestern University
Introduction to Clinical Medicine, Course Director and Clinical Associate
Professor,   2007 - 2016
Department of Family Medicine, 250 students, Introduction to History and
Physical, SOAP notes, Vitals, Head and Neck, EENT, HEENT Lab, Newborn
Exam, HEENT H&P, Cardiovascular Exam, Injection Lecture, Injection Lab,
Respiratory Exam, Heart and Lung Lab, Abdominal Exam, Blood draw Lab, Well
Child/Adolescent Exam, Abdominal Exam, Male Genitourinary, Musculoskeletal
Exam, Neurology Exam, Musculoskeletal Lab, Pediatrics, H&P Lab, Female
Genitourinary Exam
OPTO 1770, Course Director and Associate Professor, School of Optometry
2011 - 2016

12 direct contact teach hours annually
16 hours lab supervision annually
30 total hours or course direction annually

Introduction to Multi-Disciplinary Care Lectures (annual lecture) 2009 - 2016
Health Care Institute for High School Students

Wellness Lectures conducted for Human Resources (annual lecture)
2007 - 2016

Introduction to Clinical Medicine, Course Director and Clinical Associate
Professor,   summer-2011
College of Optometry, 100 students, Introduction to History and Physical, Vitals,
Head, Neck, ENT, Injection lab, Neuro physical exam, Cardiovascular exam,
Respiratory Exam, Abdominal Exam, Well Child and Adolescent Exam
College of Pharmacy – History and Physical (annual lecture)   2008 - 2010
Biomedical Sciences - History and Physical (annual lecture)   2007 - 2009
Microbiology Lectures - Micro Made Meaningful   2007 - 2008
Pathology (annual lecture)   2007 - 2008

Texas College of Osteopathic Medicine (Master's Program)

Glut 1 and 4 Receptors	1997 - 1998
Zero Gravity Effects on Bone Density	1997 - 1998
Stroke Volume Plateau when Beta-Blocked	1997 - 1998

Clinical Teaching and Supervision
Attending Physician, Cholla Clinic, 3rd and 4th year students in clinic at all times
2011 - 2016
Attending Physician, Midwestern Multispecialty Clinic, 3rd and 4th year med
students in clinic at all times   2007 - 2011
Development of Curricula and Educational Materials
Developed curriculum for Introduction to Clinical Medicine Courses, Midwestern
University   2007 - 2011

Advising and Mentoring
Students
Advisor and Program Sponsor, Career Development in Healthcare
2019 - Present
for Student-athletes, University of Texas at Austin
Advisor, Family Medicine Residency, Dell Medical School   2018 – 1/2020
Residents and Fellows
St. Joseph Hospital and Medical Center, Chief Resident   2005 - 2006
Anaphylaxis
Blood Pressure Control
Prescription Writing and Abuse
Diabetes and Management
Sub-clinical Hypothyroidism
Most Common Sports Injuries

Faculty
Advisor, Health Outreach through Medical Education, Midwestern University
2007 - 2012
Advisor, Business Club, Midwestern University   2007 - 2012
Advisor, D.O.C.A.R.E. Club, Midwestern University   2007 - 2012

Grants
Completed
American Association of Medical Colleges   2009 - 2012

Grant for H.O.M.E. (Health Outreach through Medical Education)
Multispecialty Patient Centered Medical Home Patient Care/Education through
student run ambulatory clinics, Midwestern University

Other Active Research Activities and Clinical and Quality Improvements
Projects
Leadership and Oversight of All Quality Improvement Projects 2016 - Present
Chair, Quality and Performance Improvement Committee, CommUnityCare
Health Centers

Publications
Peer-reviewed publications
Resource availability and utilization: local versus international needs
Schalscha, A., Jan 1, 2013, In: Maryland medicine, a publication of MEDCHI,
the Maryland State Medical Society. 14, 1, p. 19-20 2 p.

Invited Presentations, Posters & Abstracts
National
6th Annual Global Health Conference,   01/20/2017
Health of the World's Most Vulnerable Populations
University of Central Florida, Tampa, FL
Regional
Community Health Champions Workshop – Value Based Care 09/17/2019
Central Health

Texas House Appropriations Committee Hearing   02/18/2019
PELRP Advocacy Testimony
Community Care Collaborative Journal Club,   09/06/2018
Presentation on International Medicine

Community Health Workshop, Introduction to the Safety Net and
                                                        04/09/2018
Addressing Disparities in Mental Health
St. David's Foundation

Capstone Panel, McCombs School of Business   02/13/2018

Patient Engagement and Community Based Research,   05/01/2017
Data Intelligence in Medicine
McCombs School of Business

Community Health Workshop, Introduction to the Safety Net 04/19/2017
In Travis County
St. David's Foundation

Triple Negative Breast Cancer in Younger Women   2013
AOMA Conference Poster Presentation
Malignant Otitis Externa   2005

Academic Excellence Award
Poster Presentation
Plateau of Stroke Volume During Dynamic Exercise   1998
Texas College of Sports Medicine
First Place Award

Community Service
American Osteopathic Association, Consultant,   2017 - 2019
On Developing International Strategic Approach/Plan
DOCARE International, Guatemala: (International medical outreach
organization)

International Medical Mission Director, Guatemala	2005 – Present
Executive Director	2017 - 2019
Guatemala Clinic Director, San Andres, Guatemala	2010 - 2019
Member, Board of Directors, Guatemala	2007 - 2019
Guatemala Clinic Director, Tecpan, Guatemala	2014 - 2016

HopeFest 2012 - 2017
Bureau on International Osteopathic Medical Education & Affairs 2011 - 2016
Board of Directors - Member-at-Large
Step by Step (not-for-profit raising funds for students to participate in
international medical missions), Board of Directors – Member   2011 - 2013

UMOM/Vista Colina and CASS (Central Arizona Shelter Services), Phoenix, AZ
Faculty Advisor   2007 - 2012
Central American Medical Aide Medical Clinic, Co-Founder/Director, Ocotal,
Nicaragua   2001 - 2006

75

Appendix II
LtCol. David J. Hume, D.O.

EDUCATION
Banner University Medical Center   2006
(formerly Banner Good Samaritan Medical Center) Phoenix, Arizona
Family Medicine Residency

Midwestern University (Arizona College of Osteopathic Medicine) 2003
Glendale, Arizona
Doctor of Osteopathic Medicine

University of Miami School of Medicine   1993
Miami, Florida
Cytology Certification

State University of New York – Oswego   1991
Oswego, New York
Bachelor of Science, Business Administration

CERTIFICATIONS
American Board of Family Medicine

American College of Osteopathic Family Physicians
Arizona Board of Osteopathic Examiners in Medicine and Surgery

Drug Enforcement Agency – Controlled Substance Certificate
Advanced Cardiac Life Support (ACLS)

Basic Life Support, *Expires (BLS)*

Pediatric Advanced Life Support (PALS)

Advanced Trauma Life Support (ATLS)

HONORS and AWARDS
United States Air Force Health Professions Scholarship Program   2000
Operation Iraqi Freedom Campaign Medal, Meritorious Service Medal (x2)
Air Force Commendation Medal   2009
Operation Sentential Freedom Air Force Achievement Medal   2017

ACADEMIC APPOINTMENTS
Midwestern University, Arizona College of Osteopathic Medicine, Glendale,
AZ

Clinical Associate Professor of Family Medicine   2009 – Present
and Osteopathic Medicine

Department of Osteopathic Manipulative Medicine   2019 –   Present

    Course Director, Osteopathic Clinical Medicine II
    Second-year didactic and workshop-base clinical course
    Item writer for all testing in the 2nd year

    Course Director, Osteopathic Clinical Medicine I   2016 –2017

    First-year didactic and workshop-based clinical course

    Course Director, Osteopathic Clinical Medicine IV   2011 –2016
    Fourth-year didactic and workshop-based clinical course. Developed
    new on-line format

    Lecturer, Osteopathic clinical Medicine III   2011 –2016
    Third year didactic and workshop-based clinical course
    Developed on-line study aid for 3rd and 4th year students for clinically
    relevant Osteopathic techniques

    Lecturer and Workshop Leader   2009 –Present
    Osteopathic Clinical Medicine I, II, III, IV, V and VI
    First- and second-year longitudinal osteopathic manipulative medicine
    course

Department of Family Medicine   2009 – Present
    Lecturer, Introduction to Clinical Medicine I, II, III, IV, V and VI
    Longitudinal second-year clinical integration course

    Workshop Leader, Family Medicine Clinical Clerkship   2009 – Present
    Third-year group learning sessions during clinical clerkship

RELEVANT EXPERIENCE
<u>Work Experience</u>
Midwestern University MultiSpecialty Clinic, *Glendale, Arizona*
                                       2009 – Present
Family Physician/Associate Professor
Care for panel of patients while teaching medical students/PA
students/Optometry students and Psychology students

Luke Air Force Base, *Glendale, Arizona*   2006 – 2019
Family Physician and Flight Surgeon – Retired in 2019 after 27 years of service
Full panel of patients while in family medicine and cared for our warrior pilots
while in family medicine. Deployed twice (Iraq/Qatar) – Flight commander for
busiest Flight Operation Medicine Clinic in the Middle East. Combat flight
experience.

West Valley Urgent Care, *Glendale, Arizona*   2005 –2006
Family Physician
Cared for acute care patients 30-40 per shift

University of Miami, Department of Cytology, *Miami, Florida* 1992 –2005

Cyto-Technologist
Screened Pap Smears/Sputum/Urine/CSF for malignancy
Expert microscopist

Professional Memberships
American Osteopathic Association
American Academy of Family Physicians
American College of Osteopathic Family Physicians

RESEARCH ACTIVITY

David Hume D.O., C. Vanier MSV, H. Johnston MSIII. "Osteopathic Manipulative Therapy's Effects on the Autonomic Nervous System and Anxiety"

Poster Presentations (Peer-reviewed)

Patel, Paavan, Catherine Vanier, Mary Platt, **David J. Hume, D.O.**, Katherine Worden, D.O. *Smile! A Successful Case of OMT for Facial Nerve Palsey.* Presentation to the American Association of Osteopathy Annual Meeting, April 2014, Denver, CO.

Work in Progress

Hume, David and Mark Speicher. "The relationship between tattoos, smoking, and other risk-taking behaviors."

SERVICE
University and College Committee Appointments

Midwestern University, *Rank and Tenure Committee*	*2019 – 2020*
Midwestern University, *Scholarship Committee*	*2018 – 2020*
Midwestern University, *Institutional Review Board*	*2015 – 2016*
Midwestern University, *Mental Health Task Force*	*2016 – 2017*
Midwestern University, *Service Award Committee*	*2013 – 2014*
Midwestern University, *Admissions Committee*	*2011 – 2012*
Midwestern University, *Student Faculty Liaison Committee*	*2016 – Present*
(Third and Fourth years)	*2014 – Present*
Midwestern University, Arizona College of Osteopathic Medicine, *Alumni Association, Vice President*	*2015 – Present*

Teaching

Osteopathic Medicine 1511/1522/1533 – Course Director Year 1 and 2	2016 – Present
Osteopathic Medicine 1511/1522/1533/1631/1632/1633 – Lecturer/lab preceptor	2011 – Present
CLMD 1801-1802 – Course Director	2011- 2016
CLMD 1801/1802 – Lecturer/lab preceptor	2016 - Present
OCM III – Lecturer/lab preceptor	2013 - Present
ICMD 1625 – guest lecturer	2014 - 2017
OMM Resident preceptor –	2012 - 2014

Banner Good Samaritan Family Medicine Residency
Family Medicine Small groups – Lecturer   2010 – 2017

Advising
Midwestern University, Arizona College of Osteopathic Medicine, 2010 - Present
Association of Military Osteopathic Physicians and Surgeons,
Faculty Moderator
Midwestern University, Arizona College of Osteopathic Medicine, 2011 - Present
Business of Medicine Club, Faculty Moderator
Midwestern University, *Health Outreach Medical Education (HOME),*
                                                    2009 - Present
Faculty Supervisor for this student-run free health clinic

Community Service
City Serve Arizona, *HopeFest*   2011 – Present
Physician volunteer and medical student supervisor for this event that
serves 20,000 of the neediest from the Phoenix area
Health Outreach Medical Education (H.O.M.E)   2014 - Present
Volunteer Physician and student preceptor for homeless clinics
in the greater Phoenix region

Military Service
United States Army Reserve – Medical Laboratory Specialist 1986 – 1994
Highest rank of specialist
United States Air Force - Family Medicine Physician   2000 – 2009
Highest rank of Major
United States Air Force Reserve - Flight Surgeon   2009 – 2019
     Highest rank of Lieutenant Colonel

CONFERENCES and CONTINUING EDUCATION

Conference Participant
AOA (American Osteopathic Association)   2012, 2013, 2016
AAFP (American Academy of Family Physicians)   2013
AOMA (Arizona Osteopathic Medical Association)   2014
MER (Medical Education Resources)   2013 – 2018

www.ingramcontent.com/pod-product-compliance
Lightning Source LLC
Chambersburg PA
CBHW020158200326
41521CB00006B/425